# *Runner's World*

## HEALTH CLUB BOOK

# Runner's World
# HEALTH CLUB BOOK

by David A. Francko

**Runner's World Books**

**Library of Congress Cataloging in Publication Data**


Francko, David A.
    Runner's world  health club book.
    (Instructional book/Runner's World Books;8)

    I. Physical fitness centers. 2. Physical education
    and training. I.Runners world. II. Title III. Title:
    Health club book.
GV481.F7      613.7'1      81-23511
ISBN 0-89037-177-6      AACR2

# Contents

# Acknowledgments

The following individuals have been instrumental in the presentation of exercises for the book: Jeff Reinking, photographer; Kathleen Williams, model; Steve Henderson, model in the free weight and stretching exercises, who is an instructor at the Los Altos Athletic Club in Los Altos, California, and Patrick Oehlsen, model for the Nautilus machine exercises, who is an instructor at the S.M.A.R.T. clinic fitness center in Cupertino, California.

Special thanks also goes to the Decathlon Club, a professional health/business club in Santa Clara, California, and Beverly Trefry, Decathlon Club public information director, for the use of their facilities. We also extend our thanks to the S.M.A.R.T. clinic fitness center and George Oehlsen, fitness lab director, for the use of their Nautilus machines and facility.

We would also like to thank Jerome B. Kahn, president of the International Physical Fitness Association, for his thoughtful consideration in allowing us to publish the IPFA membership list.

# Introduction

Why work out in a gym? Because gymwork, which includes both progressive-resistance and aerobic techniques, is the most efficient and time-effective way to get the entire body into condition and improve sports performance. Gymwork develops all facets of fitness, including those that are underdeveloped by various sport training regimens. Training regimens in the gym can be tailored for either the most sedentary individual or the Olympic athlete, in virtually any sport. Whatever goals you have set for yourself, whatever your favorite sport, whether you want to run a marathon or simply lose some unwanted weight, you can benefit from a comprehensive workout program in a gym.

However, potential workout locations vary widely in facilities and quality, so you must learn to evaluate a potential commercial health club. Ask yourself these questions: What types of equipment do I need and how do I use that which is provided at the gym I join? What are some pitfalls to avoid when choosing and using a commercial gym? What types of programs should I be following to achieve my fitness goals or improve performance in my favorite sport? How can I modify my diet to compliment my training? How can I assess my overall fitness and measure my progress? Too often these questions are left unanswered in the minds of health club members. And, too often those staffing gyms are not sufficiently trained to be able to answer your questions. To get the most out of the gym or health club experience, you need to become your own "expert" on the best strategy to meet your needs and achieve your goals.

This book shows you how to become such an expert. It will start you on the right gym program and keep you going in the right direction no matter how far you advance. It contains specific information and programs for becoming more proficient at certain sports, but it is equally useful if you're interested in the health club experience simply as a means to get into shape and lose a little weight. Male or female, fat or thin, you'll soon be an expert in the use of commercial health clubs, gyms, spas, and YMCAs, while realizing individual health goals. You will learn what to include in a comprehensive fitness program, what pitfalls to avoid in selecting and using a gym, and in general, to make the gym fitness program much more enjoyable and effective, whatever your level of ability.

# 1

# Why Work Out in a Gym?

Why work out? This question will be the basis for determining your future needs and goals. You need a goal like everyone else when starting out on a new enterprise and an exercise program is no exception. After all, why should you expend a great deal of time and effort if all you will have to show for it is a bunch of sore muscles? Furthermore, why work out in a gym; what advantages, if any, does gymwork have over running, tennis, racquetball, or the like? The question of gymwork versus other sports regimens will be dealt with later, but first a rationale for exercising will be established.

First, and foremost, a regular exercise program leads to definite and important health benefits. Americans have been accused by our own fitness authorities of being the most sedentary civilization in the world. They continually bombard us with statistics that show both men and women in this country are significantly heavier and more out of shape than their counterparts of a generation ago. However, in the last decade or so Americans have become more health conscious, and increasing numbers of adults have begun participating in programs of regular, vigorous exercise. Not coincidentally, during the last several years, deaths from degenerative cardiovascular disease have declined among the middle-aged adult population. Although some scientists remain skeptical, convincing evidence showing that regular, vigorous exercise strengthens the cardiovascular system is fast accumulating. A strong cardiovascular system lessens the chance for having a degenerative disease.

Nationwide studies have been conducted on groups of men and women to determine lifestyle factors that might lead to degenerative heart disease. Cigarette smoking, for example, has been linked to the development of lung cancer. Degenerative heart disease has been attributed to poor cardiovascular fitness and appears to be one of the most important risk factors. Long-term studies show that those who reported exercising regularly—defined as burning more than 2000 calories per week in any vigorous exercise program—had much lower incidences of cardiovascular disease than their sedentary counterparts. Overweight and, of course, smoking cigarettes have been proven to increase the risk of heart attacks at an early age. Importantly, many individuals participating in long-term correlative studies on the health benefits of exercise reported that they lost weight without dieting or stopped smoking shortly after beginning their exercise program. In comparisons with sedentary and physically active people, researchers have noted that the active group is almost always significantly leaner and much less likely to pursue detrimental health habits such as smoking or excessive drinking. While many scientists stop short of labeling exercise as a panacea for all physical ills, clearly a regular program of vigorous physical exercise can become the focal point for a more healthful lifestyle.

Many other, less tangible, benefits to being in condition are known. Those who get hooked on exercise programs find that they seem to have more energy and zip in their lives. Tasks of everyday living that used to be exhausting don't seem so difficult. The physically fit sleep better and overall have a more positive outlook on life. This energetic mood has a physiological explanation. A well-conditioned body is more efficient in the transduction of energy, in movement, and more resistant to all diseases. Furthermore, the person who loses weight through a comprehensive program of exercise and diet will feel and be more efficient because he weighs less.

Exercise and the resulting improvements in body physique will also help improve your self-image. Your self-perceptions are fundamentally important to your happiness. A poor self-image can be like an albatross around your neck—it drags you down continuously, making life much less pleasant. When you look at yourself in the mirror, are you happy with what you see? When you try on a swimsuit, a new jacket or a dress, does your self-image please or disappoint you. The subject here is *not* vanity. If you're not happy with yourself you'll probably be hard to get along with. Then how can you expect others to like you? Not surprisingly, most people when asked the main reason they started an exercise program, responded that they wanted to look better. There is nothing wrong with this approach to exercising. After all, if you start exercising to look great in a swimsuit and happen to get in great shape as a result, so much the better.

A number of very important reasons for working out have been described—health benefits that are both real and tangible. Additionally, if you really want to improve your physical health and heighten your self-image, losing weight is not enough. Your body muscles must be developed to possess pleasing contours and to function efficiently. The noble goal of getting in shape requires a unified approach for success and there are no shortcut methods or miracle programs in the fitness world. There is only hard work and attention to fundamentals.

Whatever your present condition, whether you are overweight, underweight, or have not exercised in twenty years, you can still make enormous changes in the way your body looks and functions. Your body remains an amazing piece of machinery despite those years of abuse and misuse. Unlike man-made machines, which wear out with use, the human body adapts to increasing workloads and comes back stronger than before. So it's never too late to get into shape.

You will learn what fitness really means and how you can start a unified program to achieve it. If you are already an athlete, you can learn to improve performance in your favorite sport. Total fitness is comprised of several distinct components. A single physical activity is unlikely to develop all of these individual components. Regardless of your reasons for training or what sport interests you, a unified gym program is the best way to achieve your fitness goals.

## WHAT IS "FITNESS"?

What comprises the fitness state? A fit individual looks good, but that is only part of the story. A person who looks good may or may not be fit. A beauty queen, for example, may be a beautiful person in the classical sense of the word, but might also be totally unfit. She may have poor muscle tone and a sedentary cardiovascular system. What to look for in total fitness are these four equally important components: (1) leanness, (2) flexibility, (3) physical strength, (4) cardiovascular fitness. If any one of these components is underdeveloped, complete fitness will not be present. This is a major problem because many physical fitness activities do not develop all four fitness components equally. For instance, you can become highly proficient at yoga, which results in a high degree of flexibility. Yoga exercises, however, will not make you lean or strong, nor will they improve cardiovascular efficiency. Similarly, distance running is a superlative cardiovascular exercise that is also highly effective in reducing body fat levels. Running does little, however, to strengthen the abdominal or upper-body musculature. Recent physiological and kinesiological studies on long-distance runners demonstrate that these individuals are often below average in abdominal and upper-body strength. It has also been demonstrated that long-distance runners can improve their times in competitive events through gym training, which strengthens their upper body without adding needless bulk. Thus, regardless of why you want to get into shape, or what type of sport interests you, your total fitness program must be designed to develop all four components of fitness.

The fact that a gym program develops the four components of fitness equally makes it the ideal physical activity for both the novice or experienced athlete. And gymwork can be tailored to meet the needs of athletes in almost any sport.

A comprehensive gym program contains two major components: progressive resistance exercises and aerobic exercises. Within these constraints there is an almost unlimited range of variations. By combining techniques that increase both strength and muscular endurance, progressive resistance exercises common to gymwork directly increase the fitness and improve the function of the body's skeletal muscles. Aerobic techniques improve cardiovascular capacity, allowing the body to transport and use oxygen more efficiently. Together, both strategies reduce body fat and increase flexibility. The comprehensive gym program, thus, represents a unified approach to fitness and athletic proficiency. Once you have mastered the basic programs, you will have learned enough about your body to tailor your continued progress to your specific goals.

## PROGRESSIVE RESISTANCE:
## THE PATH TO OPTIMAL FITNESS

What are "progressive resistance" exercises and why are they so important to an effective gym program? To answer this question you need to understand how the human body adapts to the demands placed on it by an exercise program. First, body muscles will not develop unless they are used with continually increasing demands. All muscles work in one way or another, to oppose the force of gravity, thus moving the body. Muscle contraction forces are caused by a shortening of the fibers that comprise the muscle. As a result, the total force a muscle can exert is a function both of the range of contractive motion and the sum of muscle fibers called into action by a given load. When the maximum number of muscle fibers has been called into action, the muscle then contracts with its total potential force. Nerve impulses are responsible for the activation of muscle fibers, a phenomenon termed *recruitment*. By increasing the load placed on a given muscle, you will also increase the number of muscle fibers recruited into contraction.

This means that to increase muscle strength you must present muscle groups being exercised with sufficient stimuli to recruit nearly all of their fibers. And the stress must be of such intensity to cause the muscle to functionally overload. That is, the body must be "made to realize" that it cannot accommodate the workloads being imposed unless it increases its efficiency. In the past it was believed that increasing efficiency was garnered by enlarging individual muscle fibers, so that more power could be generated with each contraction. It has since been learned that in addition to increasing the size of individual fibers, muscle hypertrophy (growth) also occurs by the synthesis of new fibers. Thus, the trained muscle strengthens through the addition of new fibers as well as by increases in the size and contractile power of previously existing fibers.

Experts know that if you do ten push-ups per day every day for a year, you will still only be able to do about ten push-ups after a year's training. The body adapts to steady-state workloads, and does not increase its potential to do more work unless the workload is increased. If you start out doing ten push-ups, and increase that number by one each week, you will be able to do markedly more than ten push-ups at the end of a year's training. This principle of increasing the quantity or duration of a given exercise is known as *adaptation* and *overload*. You increase the workload gradually by adding more pushups every week and you give your body recuperative rest between workouts. Given a rest, the body is allowed to adapt to the increased workload and come back from each workout a little stronger.

Renowned exercise physiologist Dr. Lawrence Golding has put this principle into words rather elegantly by making a comparison between the human body and a machine: If you have a ten-horsepower motor and you put a twelve-horsepower load on it, you will burn out the motor; if you have a ten-horsepower body and put a twelve horsepower load on it, you will develop a twelve-horsepower body. Golding's thinking can be applied readily to the gym. In progressive resistance exercises, progressively more difficult stimuli (heavier weights or more repetitions) are placed on the muscle groups being trained. The muscle group must be allowed to recuperate and adapt physiologically to the present level of stress. In the next workout, the stress is increased slightly, and during the subsequent recuperation the body again adapts, this time to an even higher fitness level than before.

Progressive resistance exercises also affect other physiological and anatomical properties of muscle tissue, but first muscle fiber types must be explained. Muscle fibers are divided into slow- and fast-twitch groups. Fast-twitch fibers are physiologically designed for rapid, short bursts of contraction. They are fatigued rapidly by the end-products of metabolism, such as lactic acid, but are essential for rapid movements, like sprinting. Slow-twitch fibers, in contrast, are designed to be efficient for long periods of time during contraction. They are therefore important for endurance events. Slow-twitch muscle fibers are more efficient at metabolizing the waste products of muscular contraction, and are accordingly much more difficult to fatigue. These two types of fibers are not necessarily present in equal numbers in a given muscle group. Some individuals are genetically predisposed to having a pre-dominance of one type of fiber. Sprinters are successful at their sport because they have mostly fast-twitch fibers in their legs. Similarly, top long-distance runners usually have large numbers of slow-twitch muscle fibers in their thighs and calves. While these observations are currently under intense research, it has been proven that progressive resistance techniques effectively stimulate conditioning in both types of fibers. Also, workouts can be tailored to preferentially develop one type or the other, depending on your goals.

Maximal fitness, muscular strength and endurance are developed only when the muscle group is worked over its full range of motion. That is, the training effect must include maximal contraction and full extension and relaxation. Properly done progressive resistance exercises will train the muscle over its full range of motion. This not only increases the strength of the muscle but its flexibility as well. You cannot gain flexibility by doing other resistance exercises, such as isometrics or similar movements, because they are static.

While exercising a muscle group, blood is forced into the fibers, which congests the area being worked and results in a physiological state known as the "pump." Bodybuilders have recently popularized this term, and although the type of gymwork you'll be doing is different from a typical bodybuilding program, the pump produced by you (and all other) gym program is important because it tells you that you are working the muscle sufficiently hard to produce a training effect.

Most of a person's stored fat is deposited just beneath the skin in layers of varying thickness. In the sedentary individual, large amounts of fat are also stored between and among the muscle fibers. These fat stores act as electrical insulators and non-contractile tissues, thus interfering with muscular contractions and reducing the efficiency and force of muscular work. Heavy gym training is highly effective at reducing this intermuscular and intramuscular fat.

Working out in the gym has classically been viewed as an excellent way to increase muscular strength and endurance. Until recently, to the contrary, it was thought that gymwork was not very efficient at improving the cardiovascular system. This view has proved false. Cardiovascular fitness can be achieved through rapid and intense training. Progressive resistance exercises using the large muscle groups should be performed with intensity and few rest periods. Numerous physiological studies on top bodybuilders and endurance athletes have underscored this. The bodybuilders who trained using high-intensity techniques were at least as fit cardiovascularly as the endurance athletes. While the beginning gym trainee is not expected to have the strength to get full aerobic benefit from his gym program, he will employ some classical aerobic work in the beginning programs. The progressive resistance program will be viewed as an aerobic activity, not as powerlifting. These two forms of gymwork are quite different, as are their intended results. You will develop a physiologically balanced approach to body conditioning by the programs explained here. You will not be engaging in bodybuilding as it is traditionally viewed. Your goal will be to use the integrated gym program to develop the four components of fitness in the most time-efficient manner.

## STRENGTH TRAINING AND ATHLETIC PERFORMANCE

For a long time, coaches discouraged their athletes from working out with weights. Their prevailing view was that the strength gained was not worth the loss of flexibility or agility. Coaches in endurance sports where low body weight was important thought that it was impossible to add strength without "bulking up." These views were erroneous. Strength training actually increases speed and flexibility. Progressive resistance exercises are proving valuable at reducing the incidence of sports injuries. Furthermore, athletes who have followed a regular program of gymwork during both the off-season and the competitive season generally have less severe injuries and recover more rapidly and completely from injuries they might receive.

Strength training is valuable in maintaining pre-season strength levels during the competitive season. Lean body mass, the most important criteria in athletic potential or in simply looking good, can be either increased, decreased, or held stable by a properly designed gym program. Gym programs using progressive resistance techniques can be tailored for any sport. In all sports, male and female athletes are finding that comprehensive strength-training programs give them the competitive edge over their peers. Bruce Jenner, 1976 Olympic decathlon champion, and Tracy Caulkins credit strength training with their phenomenal performances. Runners like Gayle Olinekova (2:35 marathon) are pushing back the social barriers and stereotypes by using strength training as an important component of their running programs. Clearly, progressive weight training is not just for powerlifters or bodybuilders.

## GYM TRAINING BENEFITS BOTH SEXES

The view that gym training is something only men should engage in is an idea that must be debunked. This is an archaic view in the social sense and recent gains by women in the gym prove they too can gain strength. Gymwork strengthens women's muscles and helps reduce unwanted subcutaneous fat. Because women have only small amounts of the male hormone testosterone (essential for muscle development), it is extremely difficult for them to develop large muscles. The recent rise of female bodybuilding provides ample evidence that gymwork will produce a lean and beautiful female body, not a musclebound one. A woman's muscles are toned and better defined by gymwork. Gymwork will increase the woman's lean body mass without increasing total weight. Her power-to-weight ratio can be markedly improved. This power increase is especially noticeable in the muscles of the upper body, where a woman as a rule is much weaker than a man of the same size and weight. Experimental data on women involved in progressive resistance training show their typical fat loss often exceeding that of the comparable-sized male. From these data, it can be concluded that a gym program coupled with sensible diet will result in noticeable changes in the female body.

Regardless of your sex, a comprehensive gym program can easily result in overall strength gains exceeding 100 percent, and a significant loss of fat. The flexibility of a gym program allows individuals to tailor the degree of development desired.

## MYTHS AND LEGENDS ABOUT GYMS
## AND STRENGTH TRAINING

Through the long history of gym training, a number of myths and legends have developed. These half-truths and outright falsehoods will be debunked at the outset to allay any reservations you may still have about gyms and strength training.

**1) Strength training will make you musclebound.**

This is a holdover from the early days when all weight training was associated with circus strongmen. It will not happen as long as movements are carried through the muscles' full range of motion and attention is given to stretching the body after the progressive resistance workout.

**2) You will lose flexibility and agility if you work out with weights.**

Properly conducted strength training regimens actually increase agility and flexibility. Working out results in more efficient coordination of movement between allied muscle groups and allows muscles to exert force over a wider range of movement than untrained muscles.

**3) The gym is a place only for the macho male.**

As discussed in the last section, the gym is a place for anyone who wants to work to get into shape. Although there are still some insecure men out there who dislike the presence of women on the exercise floor, they are a dying breed. Furthermore, most gyms have separate male and female facilities. You need not feel out of place in a gym, regardless of your sex or your physical condition.

**4) You're a woman and strength work will develop large muscles that you don't need. You're afraid you'll lose your femininity.**

This is largely untrue. Most women do not have enough male hormones necessary for large muscles to develop. No amount of work will make them become large and unsightly. A few female bodybuilders have achieved well-defined, large musculatures, but they are the select few who enter women's competitions. Also, muscular development can be contained at any level you desire. Some women naturally have more ability to build their bodies. You are probably familiar with the stereotypic female shot putter, but these types of females are rare. Besides, most truly massive women owe much of their size to large fat deposits and not muscle. While most women can expect modest increases in muscle size, they will merely accentuate their femininity. Firm, toned muscles bereft of excessive fat deposits are sexy. As the woman loses fat and gains muscle, she often finds that the girth of body parts decreases. That's because muscle tissue is much more compact than the fat it replaces. The average out-of-shape female is short on muscle tissue so she shouldn't fear masculinization through any strength program.

**5) Your muscles will change to fat after you stop training.**

Muscle tissue is comprised of protein, which is unrelated to fat. When you stop training, muscles will gradually decrease in size, not change into fat. If you overeat after you stop training, you'll gain bulk, but if you reduce your caloric intake to compensate for your reduced activity level, you won't get fat or add bulk.

**6) Gymwork sounds too expensive and time-consuming to you.**

You first have to put some value in having good health. You'll defray the up-front costs in the long run by being a healthy person. Your need for expensive medical treatment will be reduced. Also, healthy people have lower life insurance rates and greater mental stability. You perform better under stress and on the job. That could result in a pay raise and promotion. We will look at the cost of health club membership and weigh that against setting up a home gym in later sections.

You may have to budget your time more carefully while training, but several one-hour workouts every week are enough to maintain fitness. Consider too that better health will result in more pep and less downtime due to illness. Sedentary living is what tires you out, not physical activity.

**7) Why you can't live by fad diets that boast quick, easy weight loss.**

You hear of these schemes all the time in newspapers, in magazines, and on television. Misleading ads promise to miraculously "melt away" excess weight overnight with little or no effort on the part of the participant. Quick weight loss is a fraud. Fat can be lost only when the caloric intake is insufficient to account for energy needs by the body. Consider this: Unless you are an extremely active, large male, you are unlikely to need more than 3000 calories per day. The strictest diet will reduce caloric intake to perhaps 1000 calories per day—consuming less, as in a strict fast, is dangerous. You would lose a little over one-half pound of fat per day on this regimen since a pound of fat contains about 3500 calories. Thus, a weight loss of three or four pounds per week is possible on a strict diet. Any loss of more than five pounds per week is accompanied by protein breakdown in vital muscle and organ tissue. Those who fast face this real danger. Potassium losses also occur while fasting, posing dangers to the heart.

When you begin a diet, the body metabolizes glycogen stores in the muscles and liver. Glycogen metabolism results in fluid losses of several pounds within the first few days. Thus, the "miracle" diet produces its seemingly impressive results only through water excretion. When you quit the diet, glycogen, which is necessary for proper muscular function, and its accompanying water are quickly redeposited in the body and the "lost weight" returns.

A real and permanent loss of fat is accomplished only through a sensible program that increases activity level and decreases slightly net caloric intake. You should not try to lose more than two pounds per week, which is best accomplished by increasing activity in an exercise program and cutting back at mealtime, while eliminating snacks. Rapid weight loss only makes the body think it is starving and triggers physiological changes that almost insure weight regain will reoccur.

To permanently change the way your body functions and looks, you must make permanent changes in your lifestyle. Similarly, spot reducing is also a myth. You cannot alter the shape of part of your body without working on the whole package. While it is possible to lose inches off your waist by doing sit-ups, you cannot lose fat from an isolated region. Fat is deposited over most of the body, in a pattern determined by heredity and sex hormones.

**8) You're too old or young for gymwork.**

People of any age can benefit from gymwork. Just as some very fine marathon runners are old enough to draw Social Security, so too are some bodybuilders 50 years old or older. These so-called "over-the-hill" people have one thing in common—bodies that look and function decades younger than their true chronological age.

There are a few precautions for the very young and very old. Pre-adolescent children should refrain from working with heavy weights, which may damage developing bone and tendon systems. People middle-aged or older should spend more time in warm-up activities than their younger counterparts. And they should spend less time in the gym, until their bodies have adapted to the increased workload. Anyone who has not exercised in years should consult a doctor before beginning a strenuous gym program.

**9) Strength training will hamper, not help your performance in running, tennis, etc.**

This is a particularly troublesome belief to the athlete in a sport that requires quickness and low body weight. Again, the common perception of strength work being useful only for people in sports like football, where mass is important, or in bodybuilding, where muscular size is the goal, is wrong. You must turn away from these old notions. Strength techniques using progressive resistance exercises are possible to use without body weight increases. Thus, the distance runner, tennis player, and the like, can increase his overall strength and muscular fitness using strength training while maintaining a low body weight.

Now that the fears about beginning a strength training program in a gym have been dispelled, you can move on to the self-evaluation techniques used to determine your present abilities in the four components of fitness. The synergistic relationship between the body and the mind and how it is important for success in your gym program will also be explained.

# 2

# Getting Ready: Putting Mind and Body Together

Most people are only dimly aware of how the body moves. Only when something goes wrong—a pulled muscle for example—do they realize the functional relationship between muscular action and movement. One of the benefits of gymwork is that you will quickly develop body awareness, a useful attribute no matter how strong your athletic interests.

Throughout your gymwork, you will be training your mind as well as your body. The mind, after all, makes you want to train. If the mind doesn't want to lift weights, the body won't lift them. Veteran athletes in all sports know that they have good days and bad days. The ups and downs could be because of bodily fluctuations; however, much of the phenomenon is due to the mind's constantly changing psychological state. You will need to master your mind to control these fluctuations. If you don't master your mind, you will not make satisfactory progress in any exercise program. Your days of discouragement must be overcome mentally, not physically.

The secret to mental control is to make the mind work for you, not against you. This concept sounds like something out of the Carnegie School of Positive Thinking. But famed bodybuilder Arnold Schwarzenneger tells us in his excellent book, *Arnold: The Education of a Bodybuilder,* that the mind can make or break the aspiring competitor.

How do you train the mind? First, you must listen to what your body is telling you as you exercise. For example, certain exercises you do will result in stiff and sore muscles. Remember this soreness and let it guide your future workouts. The soreness

15

indicates that you effectively trained those muscles. Make note of how you felt about the workout and the recuperation period. These are the elements of improvement and growth. In the gym, concentrate on each movement, each set. Feel the blood rush as you strain out those last few, vital repetitions.

To see yourself improve and grow, set reachable short- and long-term goals. It is fine to say to yourself, "A year from now, I want to have reduced my waist by five inches and improve my time in the mile by 30 seconds." But you also need the short-term goals that make the training grind more interesting and that spur you on to the bigger goals. Make these short-term goals realistic enough to be achievable. Nothing breeds complete success better than a number of small victories. A short-term goal might be something as basic as increasing by two the number of repetitions in your biceps curls, or weighing two pounds less by the end of the month.

Strike the phrase "I can't," from your vocabulary. Strive to improve your fitness *a little at a time.* Let your mind stay hungry for more; tease it a little bit. When you leave the gym after a hard workout to shower, you should be eagerly anticipating the next workout. To avoid emotional exhaustion, start your program slowly and progress steadily. Quantum leaps are for space travel, not strength training. Repeat to yourself, "I feel good; this isn't too bad at all; I'm ready for more." Then give yourself more, a little at a time. The aspiring trainee usually attempts too much at first. His body becomes sore and tired, he experiences mental fatigue and soon gives up.

## SELF-EVALUATION: WHERE ARE YOU NOW
## AND WHERE DO YOU WANT TO BE?

Become your own best expert on the status and function of your body. You need a clear idea of how to assess your present and future competence in the four components of fitness. The various benefits for training were discussed earlier. Now you need to develop some highly personal reasons for going into the gym and working out. Ask yourself, "What do I want to get out of it? What are my goals?" Be honest. Be specific. Honesty is one of the keys to progress. If you want to train to look better and feel terrific, your goal is a valid one. You may want to increase your leg strength so that one day you will set a record in the mile run. More power to you. Whatever your goal, set it firmly in your mind, so that you can rationalize working out on those days you don't feel like training. Exercises in self-realization are important, no matter what their application. Should you want to train to look better, have pictures of yourself taken and mark on them the areas you want improved. Make your dreams become self-fulfilling prophesy.

Develop your fitness to the level *you* find most desirable. You can use the self-evaluation techniques presented here regardless of your specific goals. Once you have achieved your goals you can maintain them indefinitely through a maintenance gym program and periodic self-evaluation.

## BODY TYPE ANALYSIS

Look closely at people around you, and you will notice that there are three basic body types or *somatotypes* in either males or females; ectomorphic, mesomorphic and endomorphic. These terms are so named for the three cell layers present in the human embryo. One cell layer dominates in the adult. In the embryo, the outer cell layer differentiates the nervous system and the skin, the middle layer into the muscles, and the inner cell layer into the internal organs. A thin person with long bones and stringy muscles is termed an *ectomorph* because his physique is dominated by elements derived from the outer or ectodermal layer. The ectomorph has difficulty gaining strength and weight, but has the ideal body type for endurance events such as long-distance running. The *endomorph* is dominated by the internal organs. An endomorphic body type is referred to by most people as "pleasingly plump." The endomorph may or may not be overweight, but the body type is definitely well-rounded. The endomorph has rather short limbs, and a thick torso. He tends to have substantial subcutaneous fat on the abdomen, arms, hips, and thighs. The endomorph must constantly monitor his weight and has difficulty in achieving muscular definition. The endomorphic body type is ideal for contact sports, especially since the endomorph is adept at gaining bulk. The *mesomorph* has the classic athletic physique: well-muscled, with broad shoulders, a narrow waist and hips, and moderate to small stores of subcutaneous fat. This body type is ideal for sports that require both strength and speed.

Your body type can be rather easily determined based on these descriptions; however, most people are a blend of the three body type characteristics. Analyze yourself honestly. Do you have a tendency toward plumpness or are you basically the string-bean type? Are you muscular but also slightly overweight?

Your body type is an inherited characteristic, so you will have to work within these personal constraints. If you are endomorphic you will always have to struggle to remain lean, just as the natural ectomorph will have to work doubly hard to increase his strength. But within these basic body types there is still a great deal of variation possible. The professional basketball player, who is almost always a natural ectomorph, can develop a very powerful and imposing physique. The natural endomorph can lose weight and increase his muscle mass to the point where he is functionally a mesomorph. Realize you have these natural tendencies and they will not deter you from improvement; you can work on the weak points of your body type.

Women tend strongly toward endomorphy. As much as 90 percent of all adult, non-athlete women fit into the endomorph classification. Women generally have about twice the subcutaneous fat stores of men, and even when fat levels are reduced, it is difficult for women to become as lean as comparably fit men. Their endomorphic fate is based on factors of evolution. Women have evolved to store fat for childbirth and the demands of caring for children. So more of the woman's body fat is "essential." In fact, if the body fat levels drop significantly, child-bearing functions like menstruation may temporarily shut down. This disruption is often reported in very lean women athletes.

## ANALYZING YOUR BODY COMPOSITION
## FAT VERSUS LEAN MASS

You probably weigh yourself periodically to see if you've gained or lost weight. What you really should want to know is how much of your weight is fat. Two people each weighing 160 pounds and of the same height, sex and age can have vastly different physiques. Analyze their body fat levels, though, and you'll find vastly different amounts of subcutaneous fat. The most important factor in body weight is the percentage of fat tissue that comprises your weight.

The excess fat you may be carrying is a burden for a number of reasons. Fat slows the muscular and circulatory system. Fat stored under the skin will hide the muscular development you are trying to achieve. Although fat is essential to the human body, both as a concentrated energy store and as insulation, most Americans have too much fat. Having the right percentage of body fat relative to lean body weight is an important fitness criteria.

Taking a rough measurement of your percentage of body fat does not require medical hardware, just a look in the mirror. Save the underwater weighing and soft tissue x-ray methods for when you are more serious and knowledgeable about your training. For now, look at your undressed body in a full-length mirror. If you are lean, you will be able to see the major muscle groups and most of the smaller muscles. Folds of flesh will not be noticeable when you bend over or twist your body. Your hips and thighs will not be dimpled or protrude. If you are a female, it is not hard to tell if you are too curvy.

We are interested in a bit more precision though. We can take advantage of the fact that much of man's fat lies directly under the skin. This fat layer can be pinched and measured. The skinfold obtained is then comprised of a double layer of fat and skin; muscle tissue cannot be pinched. A very good measure of the percentage of body fat can be obtained by averaging several of these skinfold measurements from various sites on your body.

Between your thumb and forefinger, grasp a vertical skinfold on the back of your arm, midway between your shoulder and your elbow. Record the thickness of this fold in millimeters when your arm is relaxed at your side (one inch = 25.4 millimeters). Have a partner measure the skinfold on your back, just below your shoulder blade. Then measure a vertical fold at the front of your mid-thigh area, halfway between your hip and knee joints. The final measurement is taken just above your iliac crest (hipbone) on the front side of your lower abdomen. Add these four measurements and divide by four to obtain a mean skinfold measure. In men the body fat percentage approximately equals the mean skinfold value. In women, add five to obtain the fat percentage. The value you obtain is probably correct to within plus/minus 3 percent, and is probably a bit further off if you are markedly overweight.

How does the value you obtained for yourself compare with healthy men and women and very lean athletes of both sexes? The average *healthy* adult male carries about 15-16 percent of his weight as fat tissue, while the average *healthy* woman is about 23 percent fat. The average adult male in the United States is about 25 percent fat while the average female in the general population is about 32 percent fat. A male would be clinically "fat" when his body fat percentage rises above about 19-20 percent, while the woman is considered "fat" above 30 percent. These statistics tell us a great deal about the relative fatness of the American population as a whole. Many of you need to lose a fair amount of fat for optimal function. For instance, top-flight endurance athletes of both sexes frequently have body fat percentages below 10 percent. World-class marathon runners usually test out at 7 percent or less. Optimum body fat percentages for world-class athletic performance are considerably lower than those for a reasonably fit population.

What percentage of fat should you strive for and how can you determine how much weight or fat you need to lose? Desired body fat levels depend on your goals and personal taste. If you're a woman you may look trim and slender and still have around 18 to 22 percent fat. If you go below that you should begin to look lean and hungry. Should you go as low as 10 to 13 percent fat (the figure varies between women), menstrual irregularities may develop. Elite women marathon runners routinely have body fat levels below 10 percent without showing detrimental health effects, as do female bodybuilders. The choice is yours. If you are a man you should have a fat level below 10 to 12 percent, or lower for participating in sports that demand low body weight. You can look very fit when your fat level is 15 percent or less.

Use your body fat percentage in calculating how much of your present weight is fat to determine how much fat you need to lose to reach your desired level. Subtract your weight in fat from your total weight to get your lean body weight. Then add whatever fat percentage you desire to this lean body weight. The result is the desired weight based on a given percentage of body fat. However, a routine skinfold assessment is much more desirable because you will be gaining lean body mass from your gym program. Thus, you may find that while your weight remains relatively stable, your body fat content decreases as fitness develops.

## ASSESSING STRENGTH AND FLEXIBILITY

Strength and flexibility are often erroneously assumed to be mutually exclusive goals. The gym programs here will improve your ability in both areas.

To assess your overall flexibility, sit on the floor with your legs straight and in front of you, parallel and close together. Take a coin or other small object and hold it in the fingers of one hand. Now bend forward at the waist and stretch the coin-held arm as far in front of you between your legs as you can. Put the coin down there. Then measure how far from the edge of the heels you placed the coin. You have good trunk and leg flexibility if you were able to place the coin at least two inches in front of your heels without bending your knees.

Try this test for arm and shoulder flexibility. Reach around your back above the waist with one arm. With the other arm reach over the shoulder blade area. If you're a highly flexible person you will be able to clasp the fingers of each of your hands together behind the back. You should at least be able to touch your fingertips to pass this test. If you are unable to pass either of these tests, you need to improve your flexibility.

Without using gym equipment, your overall muscular strength can be tested by doing the old standby, *push-ups*. Push-ups are excellent exercises for gauging upper body strength, as well as the abdomen and leg muscles. Keep the body straight and *stiff*, as you push yourself off the floor with your arms at shoulder width until they are fully extended. Then gradually lower yourself to the floor until your chest touches the floor. If you are a woman your push-up is slightly different for this test. Support the weight of the lower body on the knees rather than the feet. Your knees will rest on the floor throughout the push-up. If you can do thirty push-ups you have good upper body strength. If you can do twenty you're a shade above average. A strong athlete with good endurance should be able to do at least fifty push-ups and maintain form. Many women will be surprised to find twenty push-ups a challenge, even those who are currently participating in a sports program.

The bent-knee sit-up is a good exercise to assess the strength and endurance of the abdominal musculature. Have someone hold your feet or anchor them yourself under some heavy furniture. Keep your knees bent to reduce strain on the lower back muscles. You should be able to do at least thirty sit-ups without rest. A highly fit man or woman can do at least a hundred without rest.

These exercises will be in the comprehensive gym program as well, so you can measure your progress as your fitness improves. Remember, cheating only hurts you.

Gym training is non-competitive. You should not work out or train to compete with others, only to improve yourself. Don't get into "macho" games where you show how strong you really are because such activity invites injury. Exercising should be looked at as a process of self-improvement, not self-aggrandizement.

The mirror is a valuable tool in gym training. Use it to monitor your form while doing exercises, much as a runner uses a stopwatch to judge pace. Make it a habit. Perhaps you have been in a gym with mirrors or seen pictures of weight-training athletes working out in gyms that have them lining all the walls. They are not being narcissistic by watching themselves in mirrors. Mirrors are training aids. Whenever or wherever you work out, you should have a mirror available. One of the best indications of your overall condition is the critical examination of your reflected image. Visual progress that is observed in the mirror can be a powerful, positive stimulus. The best tonic for mental reinforcement in strength training is seeing the evolvement of your physique to a well-defined musculature.

## CARDIOVASCULAR CONDITION ASSESSMENT

Cardiovascular efficiency can be measured in two ways: the Cooper Run/Walk Test and the Step Test. The Run/Walk Test is done on a track or other accurately measured course. For the Step Test, you need a bench or sturdy chair about eighteen inches high and a stopwatch or a watch with a second hand.

The Cooper Run/Walk Test was developed by Dr. Kenneth Cooper and first appeared in his best-selling book *Aerobics*. You are to cover as much ground as possible in twelve minutes. The farther you go in twelve minutes, the higher your cardiovascular fitness rating. Cover as much ground as you can but don't overextend yourself. This is not a race. Running 1.75 miles or more rates the highest or "excellent" category; 1.5 miles is considered good, while 1.25-1.5 miles rates "acceptable."

The Step Test can be taken indoors and is similar to the more scientific treadmill stress test. Place a bench in front of you. Now step onto the bench with one foot (as though walking up a stairway), alternating feet. Do this at a rate of two steps per second (or one right-foot/left-foot combination per second) for two minutes. After two minutes of stepping up and down, take your pulse while seated. The counting sequence is as follows:

1) 0-30 seconds after the test—locate but do not count the pulse beats.
2) 30-60 seconds after the test—count and record the number of pulse beats (from 30 to 60 seconds).
3) 60-90 seconds after the test—relocate pulse but do not count beats.
4) 90-120 seconds—count and record pulse beats (from 90 to 120 seconds).
5) 120-150 seconds—relocate but do not count pulse.
6) 150-180 seconds—count and record pulse beats (from 150 to 180 seconds).

Add up the number of pulse beats recorded. If the total is over 200, you rate below average; 200-180 rates average; 180-160 is above average; 160-140 is very good and less than 140 is excellent. The Step Test is a particularly useful cardiovascular test because it measures the ability of the body to recover to normal levels after strenuous exercise.

Cardiovascular fitness tests measure your ability to do aerobic work. "Aerobic" refers to the transfer of oxygen from your lungs to places it is needed, such as in an exercising muscle. The oxygen is then used to oxidize nutrients and produce the chemical changes necessary for movement. The greater your aerobic ability, the more efficient your body is at utilizing oxygen. Aerobic ability, or capacity, can be increased through exercise.

Before beginning your aerobic program be sure you have a clean bill of health. If you have a history of health problems you should see your physician and detail your plans before beginning a gym program. If you're young and healthy you can begin right away. If you're over 40 and healthy, you should still see your physician for a checkup.

You may want to chart your progress in these four tests during the gym training program. See a sample chart in Table 2-1. Other progress charts will be described in the book, so you might benefit by writing your personal statistics in a notebook.

| Date | Weight | Fat % | Flexibility Coin Test | Pushup/ Sit-up | Cooper Run/Walk Test | Step Test |
|------|--------|-------|------------------------|-----------------|------------------------|-----------|
| GOALS | 160 | 10-12% | 3″ | 50/70 | 1.75 miles | 140 |
| 4/1 | 184 | 23% | 0″ | 15/22 | 1.0 miles | 215 |
| 4/30 | 180 | 20% | 1″ | 25/36 | 1.2 miles | 180 |
| 5/30 | 174 | 17% | 2″ | 32/41 | 1.5 miles | 162 |
| 6/30 | 167 | 14% | 2.5″ | 40/52 | 1.6 miles | 150 |
| 7/30 | 162 | 11% | 3″ | 48/61 | 1.75 miles | 138 |
| 8/30 | 160 | 10% | 3.5″ | 52/66 | 1.8 miles | 133 |
| 9/30 | 159 | 10% | 3.5″ | 54/71 | 1.8 miles | 131 |

Table 2-1. A sample fitness profile

# 3

# Choosing a Health Club or Gym

You may choose between working out at home or joining a health club. Pitfalls await the unwary in either choice. For example, there are certain components necessary for a good gym and there are useless and expensive frills. But your decision should not be based solely on which gym has the best facilities, or the idea that by working at home you'll be able to accomplish more. Your overriding consideration is the place to work out where you will feel motivated and comfortable and make the best use of your time.

## THE HOME GYM—A POSSIBILITY, BUT PROBLEMS ABOUND

A basic home gym calls for this minimum of equipment:
1) a barbell set, with at least 110 lb. of weight to start, and with the capacity to add more weights, up to 250 lb. or more.
2) a pair of dumbbells, each with the capacity to hold at least 50 lb. of weights (you can buy weight sets that have both the barbell and dumbbell bars and collars and a set of interchangeable weight plates).
3) a good weightlifting bench, strong enough for rigorous use, and capable of being adjusted for many different exercises.
4) a chin-up bar.
5) an inclined board for sit-ups (optional, but very useful).
Other equipment may be luxury. You can get a proper workout with these five items; however, a jump rope to do cardiovascular work and warmups would come in handy, unless you would rather

jog or swim. You can buy a good set of weights, including dumb-bells, a barbell and 110 lb. of weights for about thirty dollars in most sporting goods stores or large stores' sports departments. Consider buying the vinyl-coated weights if you are trying to avoid scratched floors or making noise. Otherwise, a plain steel set is cheaper and preferable, because it has flat plates that do not take up as much room on the bar as the vinyl-coated variety. This will become an important consideration later on when you're stronger and can lift heavier weights. If you're interested in a quality invest-ment buy an Olympic weight set. The Olympic set has these ad-vantages over cheaper models: heavier weights, a longer bar and weight plates calibrated in both kilograms and pounds. The plates' wider openings where they slip on the bar make them noninter-changeable with cheaper, department store sets. A good Olympic set costs about 250 dollars for a 77 kilogram (170 lb.) set.

The basic weight bench must have an adjustable backrest and sturdy, upright supports to hold the bar. It should have attach-ments at the base for doing leg curls and extensions, and hand grips on the uprights for doing dips. This type of bench costs from $50-$150.

A chin-up bar can be bought for about ten dollars. Many exer-cises can be done on the chin-up bar and it is handy for use in doing stretches after a workout.

The slant or inclined board is a useful training aid for abdom-inal exercises. A slant board costs about fifty dollars.

If you have a history of lower back pain, you may want to in-vest in a weightlifting belt. They are wide-cut, fit snugly around the waist and add support for the small of the back. They cost from $15-$25.

The least expensive home gym setup starts at 100 dollars, al-though you should plan on spending twice that to get quality merchandise. If you decide to go the home gym route, don't try saving a few dollars and buy substandard equipment from a dis-count store. It will not last long and some components may break and cause injury.

If there are no space limitations where you live there are several advantages to the home gym. First, the initial purchase of your equipment is the only real cost you will incur. Health clubs have annual fees. Second, you eliminate travel time between home and the gym. Third, peer pressure that might push you into doing the wrong kind of training is absent.

Training at home also has its drawbacks. Your home or apartment abounds with distractions. Your gym setup might be just around the corner from the television or the refrigerator. Your family or roommates can disrupt your workout. Motivational factors present in a gym will be absent in the home. Just as peer pressure can be your enemy it can also become your ally. Working in an environment dedicated exclusively to gymwork and having people around you with similar goals can fuel your interest level. At home this atmosphere is unavailable. You are not likely to have a training partner.

A training partner can encourage you to gut out those last few, difficult repetitions. A partner can boost your sagging spirit when your drive is flagging. He can watch you for correct style and recommend ways to improve. Married couples using the home exercise program can benefit by sharing a common experience. It is also a natural partnership. Choose a partner committed to your degree of perseverance and preferably of equal or greater strength. Good partners are obviously easy to come by if you work out in a health club.

A well-equipped health club will have much more than the basic compliment of equipment described previously. The extra apparatuses, while not essential to progress, speed up the workout by their convenience. Time is not wasted taking weight plates off one bar and putting them on another, or in moving equipment around so that you have room to do your next exercise. Health clubs also have wet and dry saunas, whirlpools, swimming pools, racquetball courts, etc., which are not available in your home. Training at home has basic advantages and disadvantages, as does the health club. But if you do choose to join a health club, the following section will tell you more about finding the right one for your needs.

## WHAT TO LOOK FOR IN A GOOD HEALTH CLUB

Personal tastes will in large measure dictate your selection of a place to work out. On the other hand, you may live in a small community where there are few options. Health clubs can be separated into three general categories: 1) commercial health clubs or spas, 2) YMCA's or municipal gyms, and 3) university or college-affiliated gyms. Commercial health clubs are privately owned and may be part of a national or international chain. Some examples are European Health Spa, Grecian Health Spa and Gold's Gym in California. Commercial health clubs may have a variety of brand equipment or may specialize, such as the Nautilus Training Centers. They emphasize Nautilus equipment.

Today it is difficult to generalize about the distinction between a "health club" and a "health spa." A few years ago, a health "club" could generally be recognized as a place with a lot of heavy-duty equipment, which catered specifically to people interested in intensive weight training and muscle building. Health "spas," on the other hand, generally catered to women interested in light, often passive exercise as a means of figure control and weight loss. The spa, then, was as much a social club as a place for exercise, and unsuitable for the person interested in serious conditioning.

In recent years these distinctions have blurred, so that it is no longer possible to distinguish between these two classes of gyms simply by their name. The prospective gym athlete should investigate all the commercial clubs and spas in the area, eliminating those places that fit the classic definition of a health "spa." You simply cannot get a comprehensive workout at a gym designed specifically for light, "namby-pamby" training.

YMCA or municipally operated gyms generally have membership fees much lower than privately owned clubs.

Most universities have excellent gyms on their campuses. They usually have low rates and long hours. However, you must be a student or have some connection with the university to gain access to their facilities. Swimming pools, saunas and ample shower/locker facilities are also common to most universities.

## COMMERCIAL GYMS

The prospective commercial health club member must be wary these days. Commercial health clubs and spas have been closing their doors with alarming frequency. It usually happens without notice, leaving thousands of members without the services they paid for. The health club market, like many businesses dealing with physical improvement, has attracted its share of quick-profit swindlers and honest proprietors lacking business skills. Poorly managed clubs share the same fate as other businesses—they will soon fail. To guard against joining a questionable or dishonest operation, ask the owner if he is affiliated with either the International Physical Fitness Association (IPFA) or the Allied Health Association (AHA). They set national standards for operation and management. National, well-known chains are not as likely to fail through poor management.

What happens if the club you join fails? If your club had affiliation with others in the area, your membership will probably transfer to one of these affiliates, with no loss of benefits. Affiliate clubs that honor transfers generally charge up to fifty dollars for the privilege. If your area was serviced by just one club, you are probably out of luck. You may have to take your case to small claims court to recover your investment, and then you still may not get all or any of it back. If, as many people do, you finance your membership through a bank, you may continue owing the remaining balance. Spa owners whose businesses fail often declare bankruptcy and that means you have a long wait to get back even part of your investment. Because some club chains have failed recently does not mean all of them are bad. There are many reliable health club chains.

Commercial health clubs are businesses and the way a club conducts its business can tell you a lot about it. That's why its recommended that you pay a trial visit to prospective clubs.

## THE IMPORTANCE OF THE TRIAL VISIT

Most commercial health clubs offer prospective members a free trial visit as a sales pitch. Take it! Visit the gym at a time when you are most likely to be using it. You want to see how the gym functions when you're most likely to use it. How crowded is it? How far is the drive and what are the traffic conditions like at the time you want to travel? Are instructors available at this time of day? Are the other facilities available, e.g., swimming pool, racquetball courts, and so on? Come prepared to do a workout. If you have a partner bring him, too. He also has to approve it.

Do not sign any registration papers on your first visit to the gym! Many commercial health clubs are known for their high-pressure sales tactics. Sales representatives who show you around will use every known pitch to get you tied into a contract before you leave. They may even promise you lower rates if you sign right there. This tactic is illegal. You should be able to get the lower rates quoted a day or two later. If you cannot, that club is probably a rip-off. If you feel as though you are being unduly pressured, walk out. A good health club doesn't need to use high-pressure tactics. It relies on its track record and reputation to make sales.

If you are still unsure after your visit that membership in a commercial health club is what you really want, or if there is only one club in your area, check the availability of a short-term trial membership. Most reputable health clubs offer this setup. Ideally a trial membership lasts long enough for you to make training progress (at least a month or more). Make sure that your short-term membership will convert to a full-term contract at a later date if you so desire.

## HEALTH CLUB AND GYM EQUIPMENT

A good health club or gym will have all the equipment needed for doing progressive resistance exercises, stretching, and aerobic work, as well as the facilities for warming down and cleaning up.

Conventional weights (barbells, dumbbells, pully systems, benches, and their racks), the Universal Gym and similar devices, and Nautilus machines, are all included in the training hardware of larger gyms.

Conventional or *free weights* are the best-known weight equipment and have been around since 1902, when Allan Calvert introduced what is the currently used weighted disk version of barbells and dumbbells. *Barbells* consist of long bars that hold discs at each end (with a hole in the center through which the bar passes), which are retained by adjustable collars, one on each end, that lock onto the bar. *Dumbbells* are shorter versions of barbells, made light and small enough to be lifted with only one hand. In a well-equipped gym you will find racks of both dumbbells and barbells with fixed weights, varying from 20 to 110 lb., and racks holding loose weight plates, and bars without weights. The loose weights are usually a combination of normal and Olympic plates, which accommodates the beginning lifter, who needs only lighter, fixed weights, and the advanced trainee, who may use several hundred pounds of weights in some exercises. The large compliment of fixed weights is intended to save time changing weights.

To utilize free weights more effectively, a variety of pulleys have been designed to take full advantage of the downward pull of gravity. They have also eliminated the danger of dropping a barbell or other loose weight.

The most common and perhaps best pulley training device is the *lat machine*. The lat machine is valuable for working the back (lat muscles, and thus its name) and shoulder muscles, in a manner similar to chin-up exercises.

The *squat rack* consists of a pair of stands that cradle a heavy barbell shoulder-high. It is used for doing squats with heavy weights that cannot be lifted using the arms alone. Runners or other athletes interested in building leg strength would find the squat rack invaluable.

*Benches* are often found with squat racks or at other exercise stations. Some varieties can be adjusted from the horizontal to a near-vertical position. A good gym should have several adjustable benches.

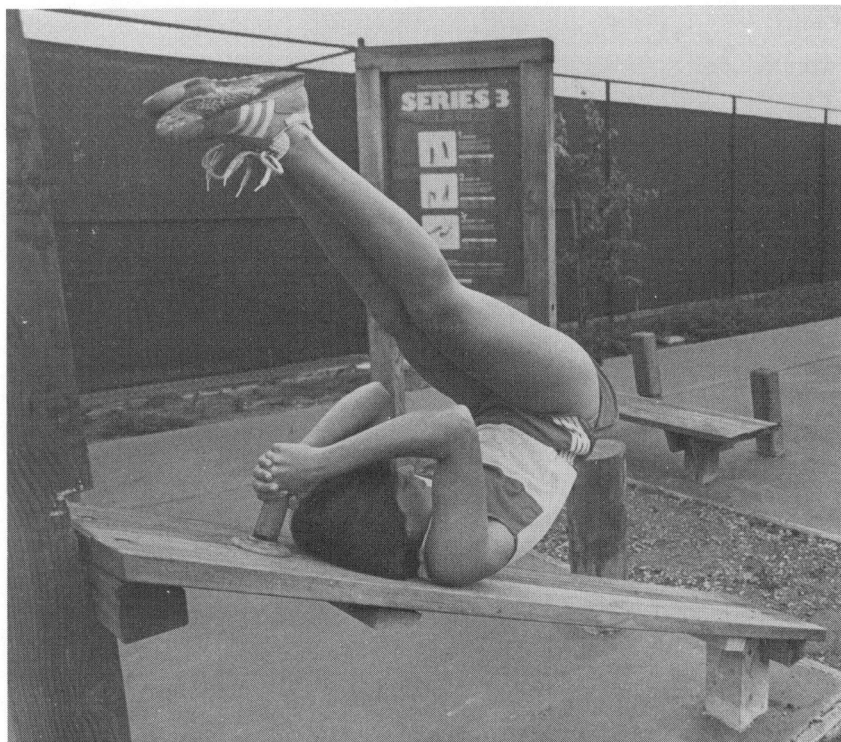

Inclined benches make sit-ups and pullovers more challenging.

A good gym might include only free weights, benches and some racks and pulleys. Free weights alone are sufficient for your needs if there are enough pieces of equipment to go around. Free weights require that you control their motion throughout the lift. They lend themselves to an almost endless variety of exercises for any part of the body. However, because of the control required to use free weights, beginners often execute their movements improperly.

*Universal Gyms* are probably the most widespread of the pulley-device machines. A Universal machine can accommodate a number of users at the same time because it has numerous stations, each for a different exercise. The weight resistance is changed quickly and easily with a movable pin that is inserted into a stack of weights, which look like wafers. The inexperienced trainee has far greater control with them than when lifting free weights. The resistance moves along a predetermined arc, which is controlled by the machine.

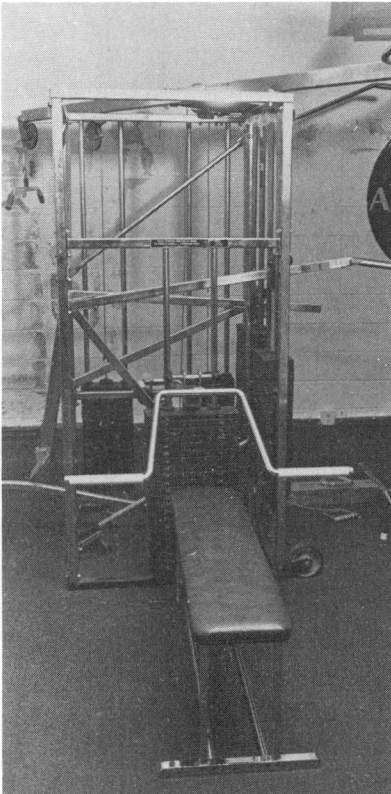

A typical Universal weight set-up.

The *Nautilus* machine is a product of today's technology. There are about twenty different machines, each of which works different muscle groups. Their popularity continues to grow, despite their high price. Certain health clubs, such as Nautilus Training Centers, use them almost exclusively. As conceived by inventor Arthur Jones, Nautilus machines offer near-perfect exercise by conquering gravity through rotary cams (pulleys). The pull of gravity is placed exactly opposite to the direction you are pulling or pushing at all times. Nautilus machines give resistance along the full range of motion, a feature not found in free weights or Universal Gyms. Muscle development through the full range of motion

A close-up look at weights on a Nautilus machine. Weights are gauged by numbers, not pounds.

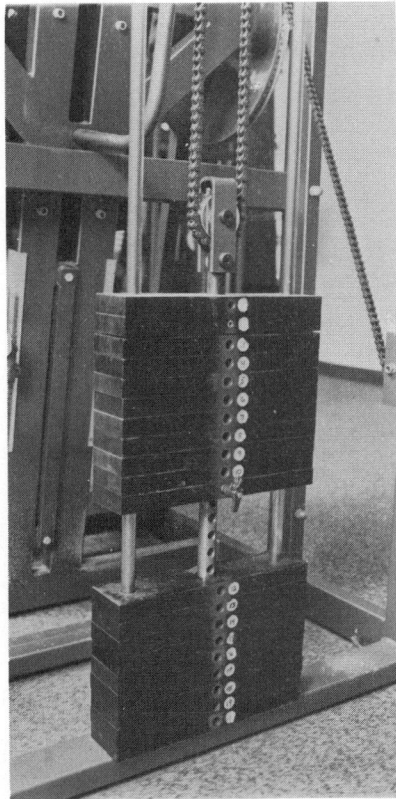

is ideal. But a controversy rages over the relative merits of free weights versus Nautilus machines. Most fitness authorities advocate a mixture of free-weight and machine work for maximum efficiency.

Aside from weightlifting equipment, look for the following in the health club: a jogging track, or at least a few stationary tread-mills or exercise bikes; bars and ballet-type stretching stations; wet and dry saunas, for unwinding after the workout; a swimming pool and a whirlpool bath. Be sure to also check the locker room and bathroom. Are there plenty of showers, sinks and benches?

The passive exercise equipment found in so-called reducing spas is excess baggage and a tipoff that this gym is not for you. Rolling machines and belt vibrators are useless. Many of the women's "fitness" centers are merely social clubs with flashy gear that has little substance. There is the erroneous feeling in many of these spas that women's exercises should somehow be more dainty than men's. Fitness, for both sexes, is attained through hard work.

An indoor running track is a definite plus for any gym. Running tracks vary widely in quality and thus potential usefulness, however, and you should be aware of some of the important facts. Because most buildings have size limitations, health club running tracks are generally small, on the order of 12 to 20 laps to the mile. In some clubs, the track is even smaller, and anything over 20 laps to the mile quickly becomes terribly boring and difficult to run on. Whatever dimension, the laps needed for commonly used running distances, the mile and the kilometer, should be clearly marked, either on the track itself or in literature available from the health club personnel.

The construction of the track is also of prime consideration.

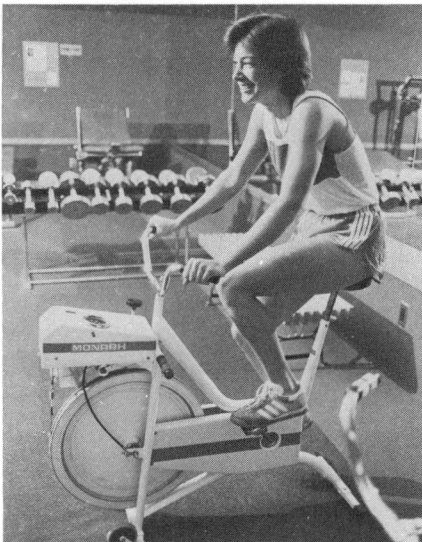

Exercise bikes are excellent for leg and lung conditioning.

The cheapest and least desirable track is an oval line painted on a concrete floor: concrete is very difficult to run on and hard on the legs. Better tracks have wood or tartan surfaces and the best tracks use this material and bank their turns.

## WHAT'S IMPORTANT AND WHAT'S NOT?

The ideal gym can be comprised largely of free weight equipment or free weights and some Universal Gym or Nautilus machines, which add variety. If you feel a swimming pool and track are important then it should have them. A good health club should have some provision for aerobic work. There are intangible factors, too, like atmosphere and personalities. When you walk in the door do you see a well-organized facility with heavy-duty equipment located for ease of use? What is the ambience of the gym? Could you get a good workout there and enjoy what you are doing? In

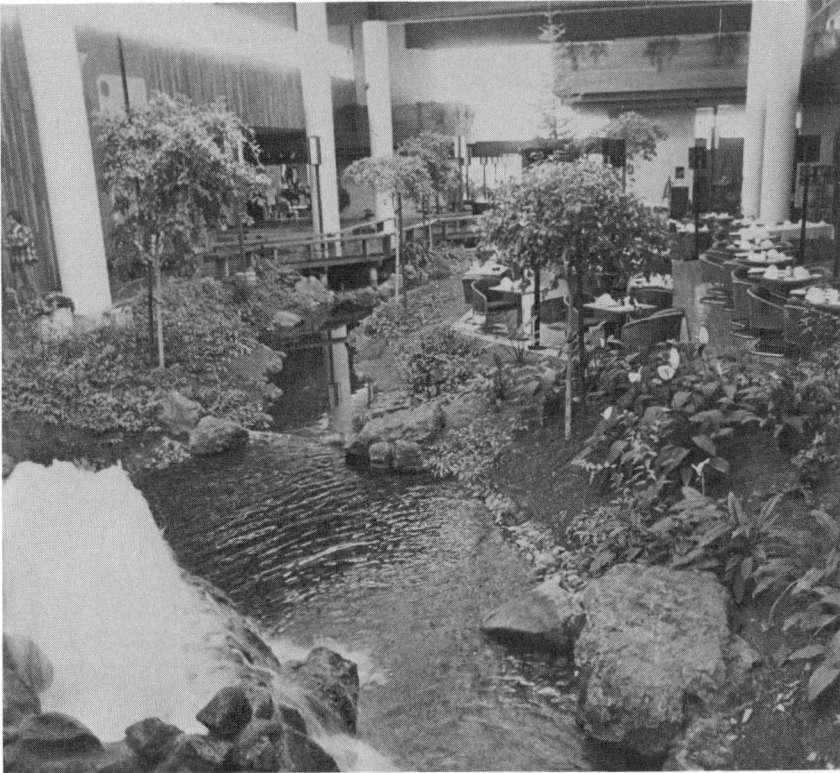

A landscaped marvel greets patrons in the lobby of the Decathlon Club in Santa Clara, California.

some gyms the members look like they're just going through the motions and not enjoying themselves. Choose a place you can identify with. Talk to some of those who are working out. Get their impressions of the place. Often, the clientele will give you more honest and unbiased information than a paid staff member. Do you find the club's personnel helpful and friendly to its members? Similarly, does the staff seem knowledgeable about what they are doing?

Environmental factors influence ambiance and should be considered. Is the training room air-conditioned or at least well-ventilated? Without proper air flow a gym can become a hot and sweaty place in the summertime. A good gym should be well-lighted. A dark gym tends to make you sluggish and sleepy. Look for full-length wall mirrors. Check the gym for cleanliness, particularly the showers and locker room. Is mold growing in the shower and sauna?

The best gym in the world will be of no value to you if it's never open. Health club operating hours are an important consideration. Most health clubs are open weekdays from about 8 a.m. until about 9 p.m., part of the day on Saturday, and are closed on Sundays and holidays. But these hours of operation can vary widely. Some gyms open early—6 a.m. is not unheard of, and many also close early. Some are not open at all on weekends. Make sure you consider hours of operation when deciding on a gym.

Gym hours are usually set by management and there is little room for negotiation. However, if enough members want the gym opened earlier or later, new hours can sometimes be worked out to everyone's satisfaction. This is one area in which commercial health clubs fare better than either university facilities or Y.M.C.A. gyms. The latter two usually offer more restricted hours of operation, especially in the early morning or in the evening, and are less amenable to compromise.

The main advantage to joining a health club is that you can take advantage of equipment and facilities that would be too large or expensive for inclusion in the home gym. As noted, good health clubs may have saunas, whirlpool baths, running tracks, swimming pools, exercise bikes, and other specialized equipment. To get the most out of these facilities, you need to know what they can and can't do for you and special cautions inherent in their use.

## CAUTIONS ABOUT SAUNAS, WHIRLPOOLS, RUNNING TRACKS

Saunas and whirlpools have been touted as miracle devices, capable of bringing fitness and health in and of themselves. While conducting your trial visit, your guide may tell the amazing benefits of these exotic water treatments. Don't be fooled by their sales pitch. There's nothing mysterious or miraculous about

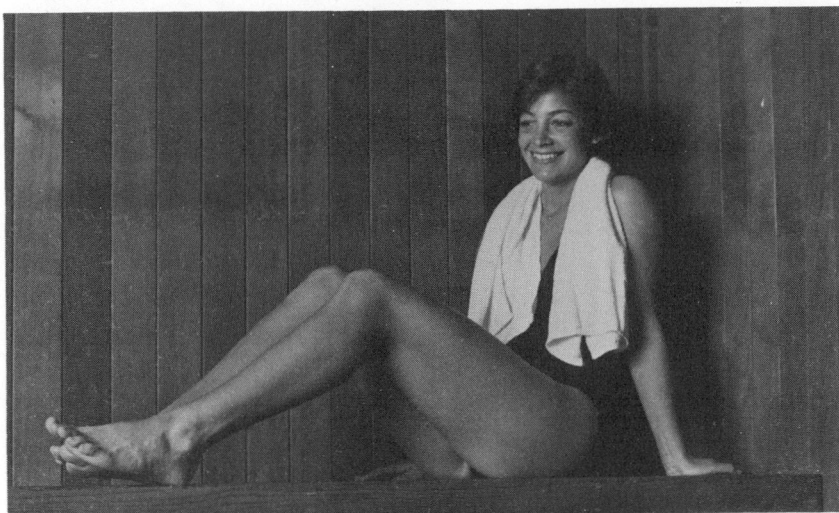

Don't spend too much time in the sauna.

saunas. A wet sauna works like a steam room, while a dry sauna is merely dry heat. They supposedly will help you lose weight and cleanse the body of impurities. Sitting in temperatures from 150-170 degrees Fahrenheit you will lose weight, but it is merely water, which is immediately replaced through fluid intake. After a tough workout, the last thing you want is more fluid loss, and excessive perspiration can produce dizziness and weakness. Additionally, the toxins produced through hard training (the metabolic waste products of muscles) are not eliminated more quickly through increased perspiration; however, the sauna effect increases peripheral circulation, as the body attempts to cool itself, which increases blood circulation and thus a more rapid elimination of metabolic wastes results.

Wet saunas are rooms lined with either redwood, cedar, or simply concrete; they develop both heat and high humidity through steam released from generators located under the benches or in a corner. Steam generation is controlled either by a manual timer, which patrons can activate, or through a thermocouple device located near the ceiling, which automatically turns on the steam when the temperature drops to a pre-set lower limit (usually about 140° F. near the ceiling). In some facilities, a eucalyptus oil base is added to water used for steam generation to open users' pores and air passages.

Dry saunas are always wood-lined and contain benches tiered from floor-level toward the ceiling. The dry heat generated in a dry sauna opens the pores and stimulates perspiration. Heat is controlled by a manual timer. A thermometer is generally found near the ceiling. Dry saunas develop temperatures between 120° F and 170°F.

If your gym has both a wet and dry sauna, spend 10 minutes in the dry sauna first and then 10 minutes or so in the wet sauna. This procedure will produce the beneficial effects of the sauna treatment without excessive overheating or dehydration. If only one kind of sauna is available, spend no more than 15 minutes or so in it before your shower. In each case, wear as little clothing as possible; if local rules allow, use the sauna in the nude. Excessive clothing inhibits the perspiration process and can lead to overheating. Never wear a sweatsuit or rubberized garment in a sauna. If you have just experienced a very hard workout in which you lost considerable water through perspiration, limit your sauna time and drink fluids before entering the sauna. Remember, the idea is to use the sauna for relaxation. Prolonged use leads to dehydration, which is detrimental to health and unwarranted.

Since both types of saunas develop rather extreme temperatures, some cautions are in order.

This is where a sauna can be dangerous. As peripheral circulation increases, blood pressure goes up and heartbeat accelerates. This may be dangerous for those with high blood pressure. Some have suffered strokes while taking a sauna. If you are middle-aged or older, or have high blood pressure, get your doctor's approval before using a sauna.

Exercise the same cautions for a whirlpool bath. Don't soak in the hot water too long or you may overheat and experience heat stroke. Deaths have occurred in whirlpools because of heat stroke. Don't jump into a cold shower immediately after leaving the sauna or whirlpool. Although this practice is widely espoused and has been made famous in ads showing Scandinavians jumping directly

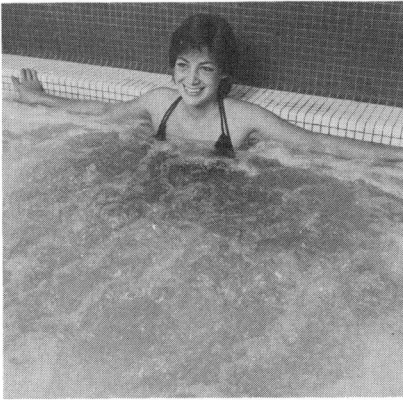

A whirlpool is a great place to rest those tired muscles.

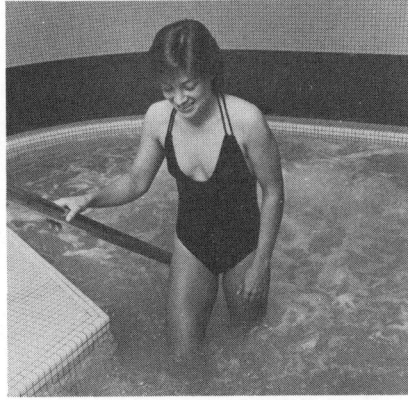

Watch your step when leaving the whirlpool. Your muscles will be relaxed.

from the sauna into an ice-lake, it is potentially dangerous. You may go into shock or have a stroke. You should gradually decrease the water temperature of your post-sauna shower.

Whirlpool baths are distinguished by heated water (usually 100° F. to 120° F.) circulating around the bather to create a massaging effect on muscle groups and joints. Water movement is created either by pumps, which jet the water around the bath, or by bubbling. The massaging action of the moving water combined with its relatively high temperature promotes increased peripheral circulation, which aids the removal of metabolic wastes from muscles and speeds healing of strained tendons, ligaments and muscles. General relaxation can be accomplished by immersing your entire body in the whirlpool. Specific body parts can also be immersed for longer periods of time in cases of injury therapy.

Because whirlpool baths recirculate heated water, there is always the danger of the bath water becoming contaminated. Whirlpools are equipped with filters to remove hair and the like, and conscientious club personnel will generally add chemicals to condition and purify the water. Much about a club can be learned from the condition of its whirlpool bath. If it is dirty, with fungus and mold growing in the area, you can be pretty sure that overall club maintenance is also slack.

Whirlpool baths are constructed either as free-standing fiberglass or wood units or are built into the floor. Water in a good whirlpool should be about three feet deep and there should be built-in seats around the periphery of the bath, placed about 1 to 1.5 feet below the water surface.

You should not spend more than about fifteen minutes totally immersed in a whirlpool, especially if you have become overheated during a tough workout. You can soak especially sore extremities for a longer time if the whirlpool is built-in or has a deck around it for you to sit or lay on. The whirlpool treatment will relax you so much that you may feel a little weak and dizzy when you get out, so take care.

A running track or swimming pool can be a valuable aid to training or can even be the main reason some people join a health club. In the northern states in particular, a year-round fitness program is difficult because of frequent bad weather. Most people find it unpleasant to run outdoors in the winter and swimmers

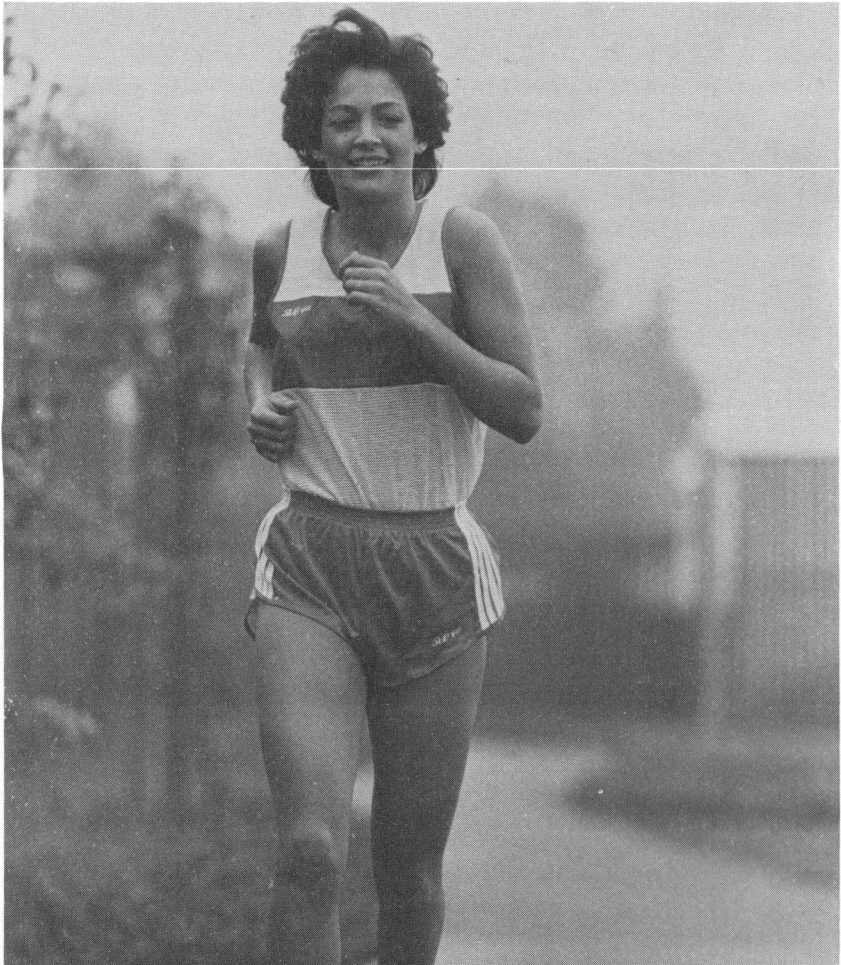

Most parcourses have a surfaced running area where you can stretch out between exercises.

must of necessity move indoors for much of the year.

Design your gym running program in the same way you would an outdoor program. Start off slowly, perhaps adding a lap each workout on a 12 lap-per-mile track until you can cover two miles or so without stopping. Then work in a combination of distance and interval training as described in programs published by running magazines like *Runner's World.* You will find that running and progressive resistance gym training make fine partners.

Swimming is a good conditioning exercise in and of itself because it works all body muscles and develops cardiovascular fitness without the pounding incurred in running. The types of indoor pools found in health clubs vary widely, from small 12 x 24 foot unheated pools without a deep end, to large, nearly Olympic-size pools with a deep end of 12 feet and diving boards. In southern states, some health clubs have outdoor pools with sunning areas. For a swimming fitness program, a pool with a length of at least 36 feet is desirable.

A swimming program usually consists of swimming laps, starting out with 400 yards (or meters if the pool is measured in metric units) and working gradually up to one mile or so. As in running, you can vary your training by alternating distance swims with faster, shorter interval swims on alternate workout days.

If you work out on a running track, don't overexert yourself. If it's very hot, cut down on your mileage or don't run at all. When you swim, be sure someone is available to rescue you in the event of cramps or injury. Work into your running and swimming slowly.

Whether swimming or running, make sure you use some of the warm-up exercises presented here and in other books before the workout, to avoid muscle injuries. Most health club pools do not employ a full-time lifeguard, so you must be extra-cautious not to exceed your swimming competence. In any health club pool, it is always best to swim with a friend to reduce the chance of a drowning.

We mentioned earlier that the condition of a whirlpool bath, especially its cleanliness, is a good indicator of the overall quality of a given health club. The condition of the swimming pool is similarly crucial. Perhaps no other piece of gym equipment has more potential for neglect than the pool area. Unless personnel are vigilant, the pool rapidly becomes fouled with pollutants from heavy use. All pool facilities are inspected regularly by local health officials and health clubs can be and have been closed for repeated sanitary violations.

If the health club you visit has neither a swimming pool nor a running track, the exercise bike becomes an especially important piece of equipment. You will use the exercise cycle for pre-workout warmups and for aerobic conditioning. Quality exercise cycles consist of a bicycle-type frame with an adjustable seat and handlebars. The pedals and sprocket are attached to a front wheel equipped with a device to increase pedaling resistance by inducing drag on the tire. Look for a speedometer/odometer and a timer on a quality bike as well as a sturdy-looking resistance unit that attaches to the wheel.

When you begin your gym program, you will "ride" the bike using only moderate resistance. Find the resistance adjusting device mounted on the frame and dial it so that pedaling at about 20 mph is fairly difficult. Then pedal the bike at about 15 mph for five minutes or until your pulse rate reaches about 130 beats per minute and you are breaking into a light sweat. Typically, you will use this whole-body warmup on the bike just after completing your warm-up stretching exercises.

To improve aerobic performance, you can work out an exercise cycle program in which the time, distance or resistance is gradually increased. The best time to work in a long "ride" is immediately following the gym program. Start out with five minutes at moderate resistance pedaling at about 15 mph; then gradually add more time or more resistance so that you keep your heart rate elevated above 130 beats per minute continuously. You can also do interval training on the exercise cycle. Try riding with high resistance at 20 mph for one mile or so, dial down the resistance and then ride one-half mile at a reduced speed; repeat the sequence of fast-slow riding several times.

Health clubs and spas will also have other types of equipment that may look impressive but really play little part in your fitness program. You may see various isometric devices—springs or tubes that stretch and work certain muscle groups. You may have seen these devices advertised in magazines or newspapers. While there is nothing wrong with isometric or "static" exercises, you are better off using weights or machines, which require movement throughout the exercise. A good fitness program develops strength along a muscle's full range of motion, while an isometric device induces strength only at the maximal contractive phase and only at the exact angle the isometric exercise is performed.

Some health clubs, especially the "spa" types will have various vibrators and rolling devices, which are throwbacks to the old reducing salon-type gym. Muscles cannot be built nor can fat be reduced by any vibrating or rolling device. You may find a vibrating belt useful to massage a strained muscle, but the action is usually far too vigorous for therapy and causes more pain than it's worth. If a health club or spa is loaded with vibrating belts and rollers, doubts should be cast about their awareness of fitness development strategies.

An even more serious problem has been introduced with the advent of the "tanning booth" in many health clubs. These booths use relatively high-intensity ultraviolet (UV) light to induce rapid production of melatonin, the skin pigment that produces a tan. While you are supposed to wear safety goggles during tanning and limit your exposure to the UV light, few people are as cautious as they should be. Excessive exposure to UV light in sunlight is known to cause premature skin wrinkling and skin cancer. It is wise to avoid tanning booths in health clubs, especially if you are fair-skinned or if you receive heavy exposure to natural sunlight in your daily life. While no one can say for sure that such "fast-tanning" booths are harmful, it is always best to err on the side of safety.

Besides the information already given about what to look for in a reliable health club, you should contact your local consumer complaint agency. It keeps a file of complaints against commercial businesses. Beware of health clubs with a large number of complaints.

## THE HEALTH CLUB CONTRACT

Health clubs' annual membership fees range from about fifty dollars in the smaller, less well-equipped clubs, to about 450 dollars in deluxe clubs with swimming pools, running tracks and the like. Health club memberships may last one month or several years. You may reduce your fee considerably through a long-term membership, but be certain you are happy with the club and that you don't plan to move in that time. If you sign up for a long-term membership and do move, a national chain or a club affiliated with the International Physical Fitness Association or the Allied

Health Association, will allow a transfer (for a small fee) to another member club, but only those within each group. The IPFA and AHA each have hundreds of facilities in the United States and in several foreign countries, but they do not recognize switches between member clubs. The IPFA requires that their affiliates pay a 500 dollar annual affiliation fee. The AHA requires no fees of their members.

Taking advantage of special offers that occur when a new facility opens is another way to save on membership fees. During the first few weeks of operation, a new club may offer memberships for as little as half-price to entice new members. Consider, though, the possibility that the new club won't make it. If you have a friend interested in health club membership, you can often get a special two-for-one membership rate, even if such a rate is not specifically advertised. Similarly, most health clubs offer add-on memberships for members of the same family, usually at significant savings. Make sure you inquire about these special features before signing a contract.

A composite sample gym contract with explanation of some specific terms is given in the Appendix.

Your contract should spell out your benefits which should include the following: the length of membership, the cost for the initial period of membership, the annual fee for the long-term contract, and a clause that states you can cancel the membership due to illness or injury. A reciprocity clause (allowing club switch in case of relocation) if available, should be included.

Most clubs unfortunately require payment in full or you might have to finance the cost of membership. Installment plans are hard to come by. Under this arrangement you have few options if the club goes out of business. Your contract is also legally binding, whether it be at a YMCA or commercial health club. If you get tired of working out and want to quit, you're out a year's membership, unless a medical problem prevents you from attending the club.

## WHAT TO LOOK FOR IN A HEALTH CLUB

1) Location: near home or work?
2) Hours of Operation: Saturday and Sunday? Evenings?
3) Equipment: Free weights; Universal Gyms; Nautilus machines; chin-up bars; ballet stretching stations; mirrors; ample incline,

decline, and regular benches; swimming pool; running track; stationary exercise bikes; running treadmill; wet or dry saunas; whirlpool baths.

4) Locker Room/Shower Facilities: Clean, roomy.

5) Paid Staff: Knowledgeable, friendly, helpful to patrons? Availability?

6) Ventilation: Air-conditioned or at least well-ventilated?

7) Costs: Annual fee; price of long-term membership; price of add-on membership; yearly maintenance fee; special offers.

8) General Ambiance: Can you get a good workout there? Do patrons seem to enjoy the gym? Is the facility clean, well-organized and roomy? Will you feel comfortable there?

9) Reliability: If a commercial health club, how long has it been in business? Is it part of a national chain or affiliated with the IPFA or AHA? What are reciprocity privileges with other spas?

10) Are all major and minor benefits spelled out? What happens if you are ill? Must you pay in full at the beginning? Do you understand all of the contract?

# 4

# Laying the Foundation for Gymwork

Before you start serious training, you must gradually adapt your body to progressive resistance exercises. This is especially true if you have never trained with weights, or if it has been more than a year since your last workout. A good foundation is just as important in gymwork as it is in other sports. You would not run a 10,000-meter race without enough training to know you can finish. Those who jump into weightlifting usually wind up with sore muscles, stiff joints and possibly an injury. This is enough to make any novice decide to quit. But the very basis of progressive resistance training is to introduce stress a little at a time, and avoid overtraining. Adaptation is the key. It will not occur if excessive stress is applied to the body too soon. The best investment you can make as a novice gym athlete, even if you already participate in another sport, is to develop a sound foundation.

## THREE GENERAL TYPES OF GYM EXERCISES

Gymwork is aimed at developing fitness in three major parts of the body: 1) the upper body, 2) the lower body, and 3) the abdominals. The muscles of these three groups work synergistically to allow movement, and the exercises you do will both develop each muscle group independently as well as coordinate the action of allied muscle groups. Refer to the illustration on muscle anatomy to familiarize yourself with the body.

Developing all three of the functional groups, as well as the cardiovascular system, is crucial even if your sport stresses one functional group over another. For example, while a sprinter may rely

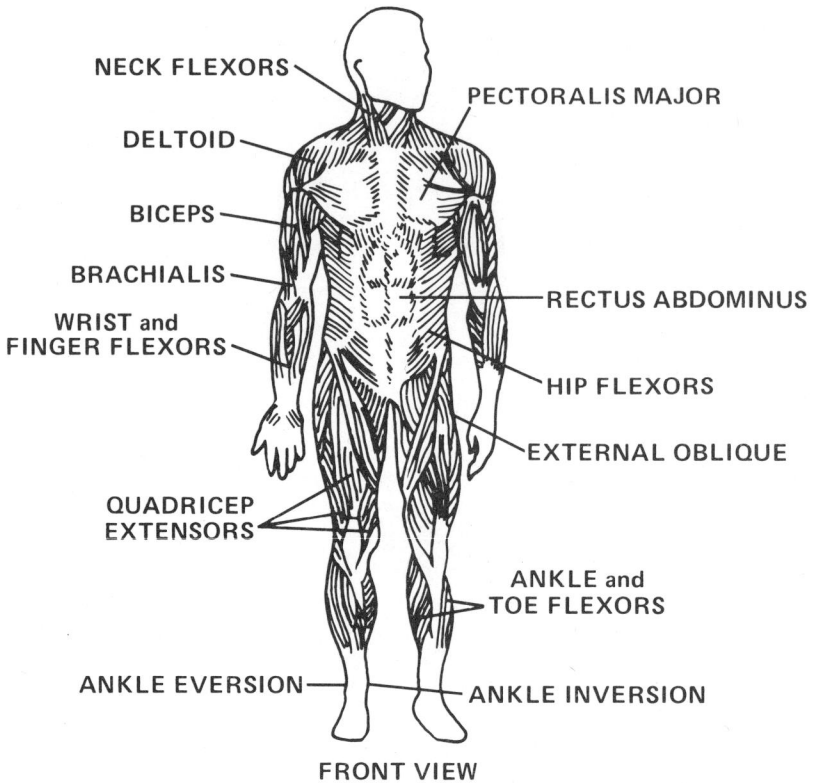

FRONT VIEW

on the quadriceps muscle of the thigh for power and speed, his performance will be hindered unless he has sufficient upper body and abdominal strength as well. Sprinters are especially prone to muscle pulls of the hamstrings because these muscles, which act antagonistically to the quadriceps, are generally not trained to the degree the quadriceps are. A functional imbalance in the power generated by the leg develops as a result and the weaker muscle group becomes prone to injury.

Most training injuries, and indeed most sports injuries in general, happen either when you overextend a poorly trained body part or spend insufficient time warming up. The *freehand exercise program* here is designed to prepare your body for the rigors of heavy training. A properly conducted freehand foundation pro-

NECK EXTENSORS

TRAPEZIUS

TERES MAJOR

LATISSIMUS DORSI

GLUTEUS MAXIMUS

HAMSTRINGS

TRICEPS

ERECTOR SPINAE

WRIST and
FINGER EXTENSORS

CALF (GASTROCNEMIUS)

SOLEUS

**BACK VIEW**

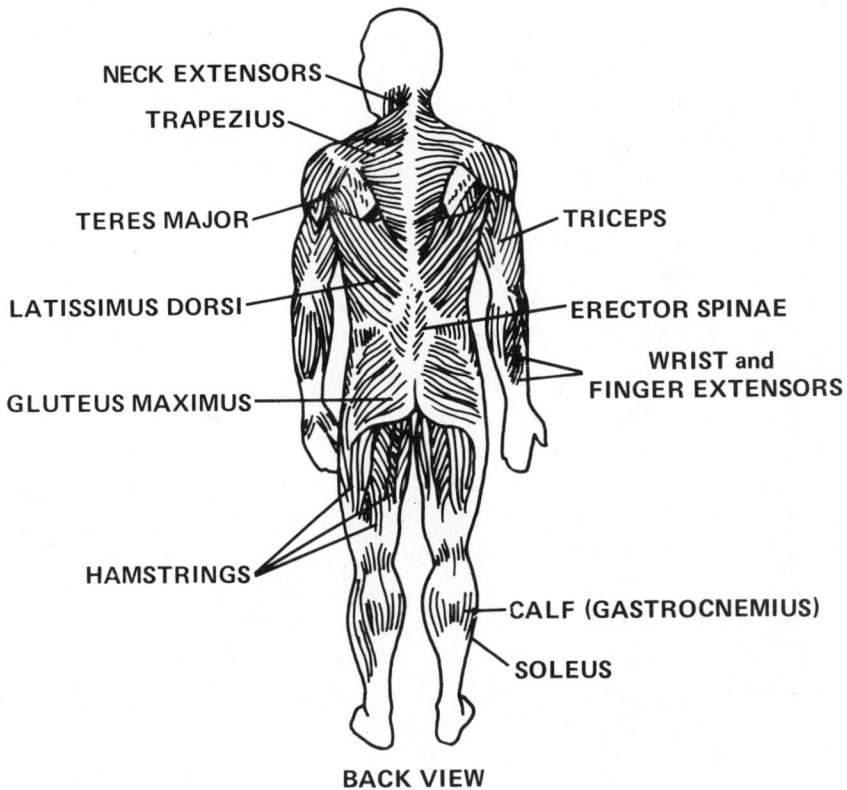

gram will work the cardiovascular system sufficiently to develop aerobic fitness. Pre- and post-workout stretching exercises are also included.

## TRAINING HINTS

In the freehand program and in the beginning gym program, you should try to work out three times a week, with at least one day of rest between workouts. The rest day is as important as the workout itself, because this is when the body adapts physiologically to the stresses placed on it. You can make progress on just two sessions a week, but your improvement will be at a slower pace.

Clothing requirements are minimal for gymwork. It should be comfortable and allow maximum freedom of movement. Wear as little as the ambient temperature will allow. If you can get away with shorts, all the better. This allows you to see the various muscle groups as you train. Many will do the opposite—hide their trouble spots and areas of weakness under layers of clothing. Exposing that flabby stomach will be a constant reminder that you still have work to do.

Avoid wearing heavy sweat clothes or the special rubber exercise suits. You may sweat a lot and lose some weight but they can be dangerous. You may suffer heat exhaustion. Weight lost will be in the form of water anyway, and quickly replaced after the workout. Instead, wear lightweight clothing. It will enhance sweat evaporation, which cools the body. The mirror will be a more effective training tool, too. Watch the muscles contract as you work and check your form as you go through the exercise motions.

Breathing properly is very important in strength training. In almost every exercise, you will inhale on the downward stage. For example, when you do a pushup, exhale as you push yourself off the floor and inhale as you lower your body. When you do a sit-up, inhale as you lie down and exhale as you raise your torso. This cadence will quickly become second nature, because the diaphragm muscles, which control breathing, will relax and contract in the same tempo as the skeletal muscles. Breathe in and out at least one time for every repetition and never hold your breath while exerting a muscle group because it can lead to a muscle pull.

You will need to tread a fine line between hard work and overtraining. Distinguishing between these two states requires that you develop increased body awareness. Injury is a sign of overtraining, as is being chronically tired, short-tempered and losing your appetite.

## KEEPING A TRAINING LOG

The freehand program lends itself well to keeping a personal training log. Most commercial gyms will issue a training workout card, which lists specific exercises, repetitions, and other important information. But it is still best to keep your own, more detailed training log to track your progress and as a means of self-evaluation.

A detailed training log will include such information as exercise routine, the number of repetitions completed, and feelings (both physical and mental) after each workout. Record areas of soreness. Periodically measure and record body dimensions such as chest, waist, thigh, calf, upper arm, and so on. Track body fat levels and body weight. The training diary will assist the development of body awareness and give you a permanent record of your progress. Graphic evidence of your progress might even amaze you. You will be able to tell which fitness aspect is working best or what body part needs more attention to increase strength. A sample training log is found in Table 4-1.

## FORMAT FOR PRESENTATION OF EXERCISES

In both the freehand exercise program and the subsequent gym programs, exercises will follow the same format. There are several key words: *Repetitions*—expressed as number. Total times each movement is completed. *Set*—a number of repetitions conducted as a group. *Movement*—another term for an exercise. *Program*—a unified group of sets of exercises, with each set comprised of a given number of repetitions. *Rep*—short for repetition.

Each exercise will be presented in the following format:

1) **Basic movement** (how to do the exercise and on what apparatus).

2) **What it does** (the specific muscle groups the exercise develops and other basic benefits).

3) **Variation on a theme** (additional ways of doing an exercise to get slightly different effects, or ways to do the same movement on another piece of equipment).

4) **Special considerations** what to look for in force of movement, breathing, pauses between repetitions or sets, etc.).

A Sample Personal Training Log/Self-Assessment Format
(program of a young male trainee)

**Week of May 5-12**

| Exercise | Reps/Sets Scheduled | Reps/Sets Completed | | |
|---|---|---|---|---|
| | | May 5 | May 7 | May 10 |
| sit-up | 15/2 | 15/2 | 16/2 | 17/2 |
| knee-ups | 10/2 | 10/2 | 10/2 | 11/2 |
| parallel dips | 4/2 | 5/2 | 5/2 | 6/2 |
| rowing between chair | 10/2 | 10/2 | 10/2 | 11/2 |
| pushups | 15/2 | 16/2 | 17/2 | 18/2 |
| lunges | 15/2 | 20/2 | 20/2 | 22/2 |
| pullups | 5/2 | 5/2 | 5/2 | 5/2 |
| calf raises | 15/2 | 15/2 | 15/2 | 15/2 |

**Notes:**

Table 4-1

May 5: Felt strong doing pushups; will try to add one rep each workout. Very sore in abdomen after doing sit-ups/knee-ups; add one more sit-up each workout this week.

May 7: Was able to do one more rep each in pushup only; abdominals still lagging. Sore in shoulders after doing pullups.

May 10: Tried to add one more rep in every exercise. Pullups still seem to be weak area, but I feel stronger each day and ready for next week's work. Seeing more definition in abdomen.

**Plans for Next Week**

Will try to add one more rep per exercise next week. Continue that strategy for two weeks or so, then go up to three sets of each exercise the following week, dropping reps down to level of May 5-12.

**Measurements (May 5)**

| Chest | Upper arm (left/right) | waist | thigh (left/right) | shoulder | calf |
|---|---|---|---|---|---|
| 38" | 13½"/14" | 34" | 22"/22¼" | 44" | 14" |

**Weight:** 181 lb.

**Body Fat:** 20%

**Flexibility:** placed coin 1¼ inches from heels; can almost touch fingers behind back.

**Step Test Pulse:** 185 beats/minute

## WARMING UP BEFORE THE WORKOUT

A good warmup is absolutely essential before any progressive resistance workout. You want to increase blood circulation through the muscles and stretch the muscles and ligaments that you will key on in the workout. An insufficient warmup is one of the prime causes of athletic injuries.

Five to ten minutes of warm-up activities will increase efficiency of the muscles. Include activities to stretch the muscles and get the pulse rate going without putting a heavy load on either the muscles or cardiovascular system. Keep up a steady pace, resting only fifteen to thirty seconds between exercises. All movements should be fluid and unforced. Gradually increase your extension, until you feel mild pain in the muscle being stretched. and hold that position a few seconds before relaxing. Bouncing is counterproductive because it activates what is called the stretch reflex mechanism. Once activated, the range of motion in the muscle group is limited.

There are hundreds of exercises that can form the basis of a good warm-up routine, some of which will be presented here, but you need not feel confined to these. *The Runner's World Yoga Book* by Jean Couch has many stretching exercises that you may use. A basic warm-up routine might include:

1) Jumping jacks: 50 repetitions
2) Lower back/hamstring stretch: 60 seconds to each side
3) Side bends/twists: 30 repetitions to each side
4) Pulling on a pole: 60 seconds to each side
5) Towel stretch: 60 seconds to each side
6) Chinning bar hang: 60 seconds
7) Calf stretch: 30 seconds each calf
8) Crossed-legs lower back/hamstring stretch: 60 seconds to each side
9) Jogging/jumping rope/stationary bike: 5 minutes or until you break into a sweat.

This program will take you 10-15 minutes, warm up all of the muscle groups and get your circulation going. If you have not worked out in a long time or are middle-aged or older, make sure you do not skimp on your warm-up time. Excessive muscle soreness will result and you increase the risk of a muscle pull or strain.

## WARM-UP EXERCISES

### Jumping Jacks

**Basic movement**: Stand with your feet together and your arms pressed at your sides. In a single, coordinated move you will spread both your legs and arms. Spring off your feet and spread your legs so that they land simultaneously about two feet apart. As you are moving your legs, simultaneously bring your arms (unbent) over your head. You may want to clap your hands. Return to your original position by simultaneously moving both legs and arms. This makes one repetition. Develop a fluid rhythm, with no stops anywhere in the movement. Coordinate the movement of arms and legs.

**What it does**: Involves all of the major skeletal muscles and gets the heart rate up to training levels.

**Variations on a theme**: The movement should be completed in about one second. Near the end of the set try speeding up the movement slightly.

**Special considerations**: Maintain an even cadence with no stops, unless you employ the above variation. If you are a beginner, you may want to start at twenty-five repetitions and work your way up.

### Lower Back/Hamstring Stretch

**Basic movement**: Spread your legs two or three feet apart while standing and lock your knees. Spread your arms straight out to your sides and parallel to the ground. From this position, bend down and with your left hand touch your right instep. Keep your knees and arms straight during the movement. Return to the starting position and repeat the movement to the opposite side. Alternate sides at a steady cadence for about two minutes.

**What it does**: This is a fine stretching exercise for the spinal erector muscles of the back and for the hamstring muscles of the back of the thigh.

**Variations on a theme**: Keep your hands on your instep for three to five seconds.

**Special considerations**: Don't bounce when reaching down to touch the instep. Go slowly; a complete left-to-right cycle should last about five seconds.

## Lower Back/Hamstring Stretch

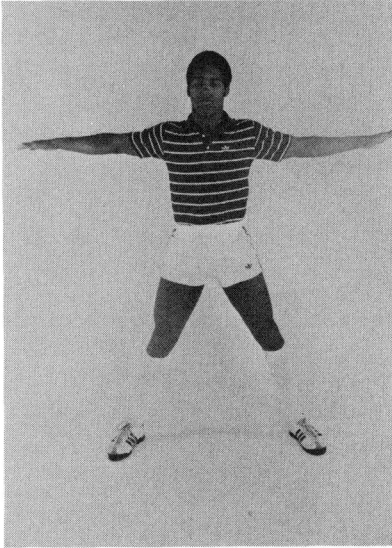

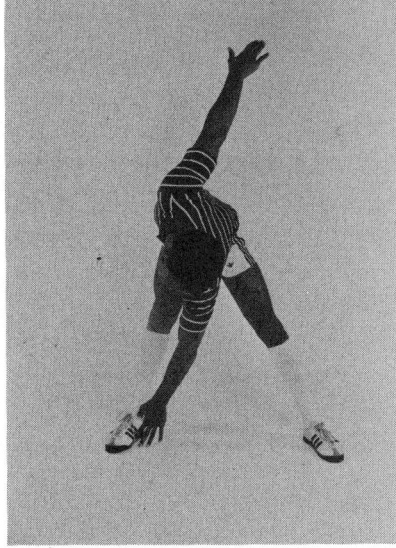

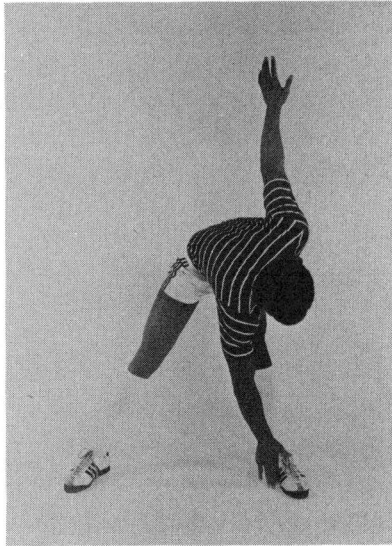

Begin the lower back/hamstring stretch with arms and hands parallel to the floor. Extend your arms straight and down to one foot, then the other.

## Side-Bends/Twists

**Basic movement**: Standing erect, place your hands on your hips. Slowly rotate your body full-circle, first to the left and then to right, bending at your waist. Hold the position of maximum stretch for a few seconds and then return to the starting position.

## Side-Bends/Twists

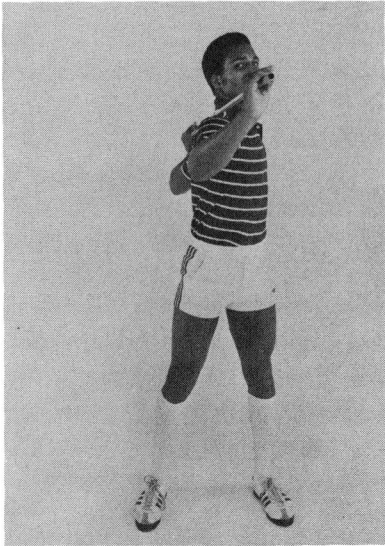

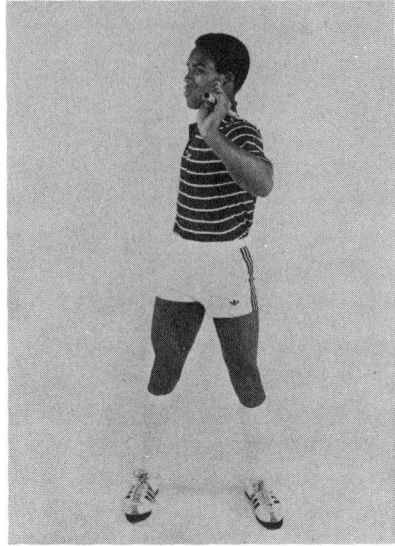

Side bends/twists can be done while standing upright or while bending at the waist. This exercise works the abdominals.

**What it does**: This movement warms up the abdominals and the oblique muscles at the sides of the waist.

**Variations on a theme**: Place a broomstick on your shoulders behind your neck, holding an end in each hand. Use the same rotating motion as in the basic movement. A broomstick variation is done from a bent-over position, where your upper body is bent at the waist and parallel to the ground. Now twist your upper body so that the end of the broomstick in your right hand touches your left instep; then touch the left end of the broomstick to your right instep.

**Special considerations**: Side-bends can be done fairly quickly. In addition to being a good warm-up activity, this exercise is effective in toning abdomen muscles. It firms up those "love handles" so many of you have on the sides of your waists. Go for the maximum stretch when you twist. When you really feel the stretch, you are also loosening your shoulder muscles and those of the upper back.

### Pole Pulling

**Basic movement**: Stand about eighteen inches away from an upright pole or bar (you can also hang on to both sides of a door handle). Grasp the pole at approximately shoulder level and interlace your fingers. Bend your knees slightly as you sink toward the floor until your back forms about a 45-degree angle with the floor. Then force your hips away from the bar, so that you feel the stretch in your back and sides of your back. Now pull yourself up until your forehead touches the bar, making sure you use the muscles of your arms and back in a slow, fluid motion, Repeat the up-and-down movement, striving for maximal stretching each time.

**What it does**: This movement stretches the latissimus dorsi muscles of the upper sides of the back. It also stretches to a lesser degree all of the other muscles of the upper back. The latissimus dorsi muscles give a V-shaped appearance to the upper torso of the trained athlete and are important for any movement involving the back muscles.

**Variation on a theme**: Twist your hips slightly at the bottom of the movement, in a back-and-forth motion. This will stretch your lats (a useful abbreviation for the latissimus dorsi) even more.

**Special considerations**: Always pause at the bottom of the movement, as you really feel the stretch in your back muscles. Make sure the movement is fluid. This is another movement where bouncing is counterproductive.

**Towel Stretch**

**Basic movement**: With your palms facing your thighs, grasp a towel or rope in front of your thighs with both hands, so that the distance between your hands is two feet greater than the width of your shoulders. Keeping your arms straight, lift them over your head and spread them as far apart as the towel or rope will allow. Then arc your right arm to the rear and down toward your side until your left arm is straight up, and its bicep resting against your left ear. Move your right arm backward, as far as you can while still keeping your elbows locked. Follow the right shoulder dislocation with a similar movement of your left arm and shoulder so that both arms are extended behind your back. Then reverse this movement, one arm at a time, until reaching the starting position again.

**What it does**: The towel stretch loosens the shoulder muscles and is good in preparing for pressing exercises that use the shoulder muscles.

**Variations on a theme**: When both arms are behind your back, pull hard on the towel or rope, so that you feel your chest muscles

## Towel Stretch

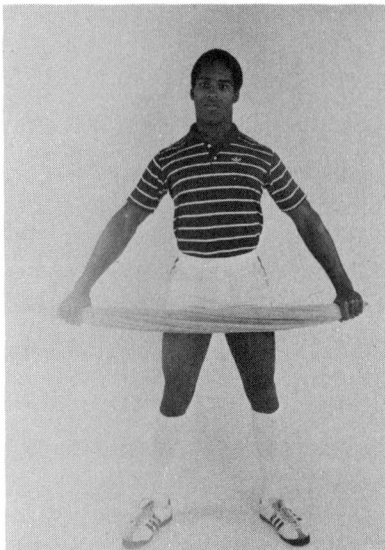

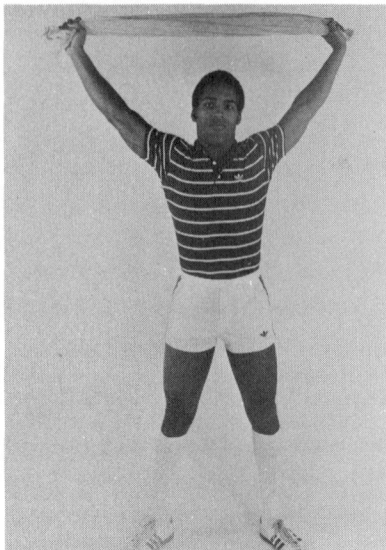

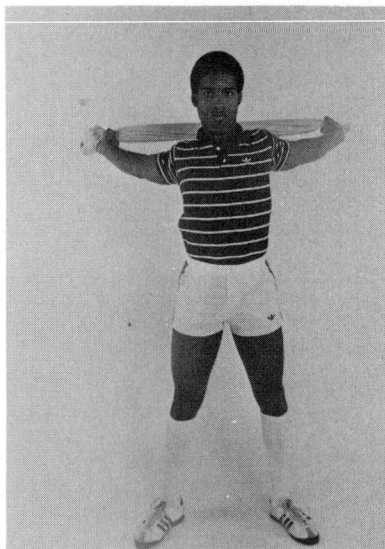

Start the towel stretch at your waist and continue the movement over your head to the back of your neck. As you gain flexibility decrease the distance between your hands.

stretching. This variation loosens and stretches the pectoral muscles of the chest as well as the serratus muscles of the chest wall.

**Special considerations:** As you become more supple, decrease the distance between your hands on the towel or rope. When you can do this movement with your hands placed at shoulder width or narrower, you will know you have superior shoulder flexibility.

### Chinning Bar Hang

**Basic movement**: If you do not have access to a chinning bar, a strong pipe suspended from the ceiling will do, provided it is sturdy enough to handle your weight. Grasp the bar with your palms facing outward and your hands placed a little farther apart than the width of your shoulders. Then simply pull your feet off the floor and hang from the bar, making no effort to counteract gravity, so that you can really feel the stretch. Try to hold this position for about thirty seconds and then repeat.

**Chinning Bar Hang**

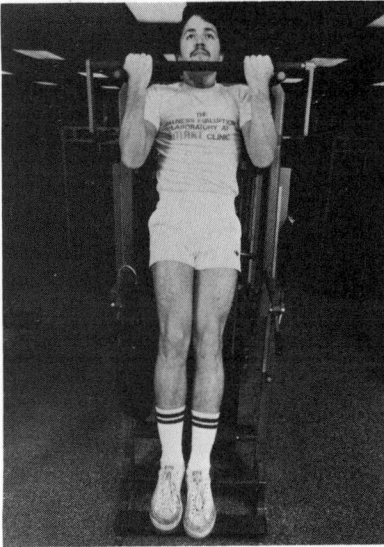

Chinning bar hangs are done on a bar, keeping the palms of the hands facing you or away from you. Chin-ups are also done from the bar hang position.

**What it does**: Hanging from the chinning bar stretches all of the muscles of the upper body.

**Variations on a theme**: Instead of placing your hands with the palms facing outward, place your palms so that they face toward you. This variation will stretch your biceps muscles that are in the front of your upper arm.

**Special considerations**: This exercise may be fatiguing, especially for women, who naturally have less upper body strength than man. Try to hang from the bar until feeling fatigued and then relax for several seconds and repeat the exercise. You will be surprised at how fast you can improve and soon you will be able to hang for thirty seconds at a time with ease. This is a warm-up activity so do not overdo this movement.

### Calf Stretch

**Basic movement**: Stand about eighteen inches away from and facing a wall, with your feet about shoulder-width apart. Place your hands on the wall in front of you, also about shoulder-width apart and chest level. Simultaneously "walk" your arms down the wall and move your feet away from the wall, keeping your body straight at all times. When your body is at about a 45-degree angle from head to feet, you will note that you are now standing on your toes. Hold this position for a few seconds. Then, moving only your ankle joints, try to force your heels to the ground while keeping your knees locked and your body straight. After each downward stretch, rise on your toes and stretch down again.

**What it does**: Calf stretching loosens the calf muscles, which are particularly prone to strain if not warmed up properly.

**Variations on a theme**: After a week or two you should be able to lower and raise the weight of your entire body using just one calf at a time. When you can do this, alternately raise and lower your weight for about thirty seconds per leg.

**Special considerations**: Calf stretching is particularly valuable for runners who will be subjecting their calf muscles to the rigors of both weight training and running. If you are prone to muscle spasms of the calf, make sure you do this movement slowly and completely.

### Crossed-Legs Lower Back/Hamstring Stretch

**Basic Movement**: This exercise is slightly more demanding than the other lower back/hamstring stretch already described, so it should be done near the end of the warmup, when your muscles are sufficiently supple. It is an excellent finishing stretch for the back and the hamstrings. Stand erect with your arms at your sides and cross your right foot over your left foot. Bend at your waist and try to touch your hands to your toes. Make sure you don't bend your knees and make this a smooth motion with no bouncing. Return to the starting position and repeat for about ten repetitions. Alternate until you have done this movement for about 60 seconds to each side.

**What it does**: Stretches the entire posterior half of the body.

**Variations on a theme**: Try to bring your hands to a position

## Crossed-Legs Hamstring Stretch

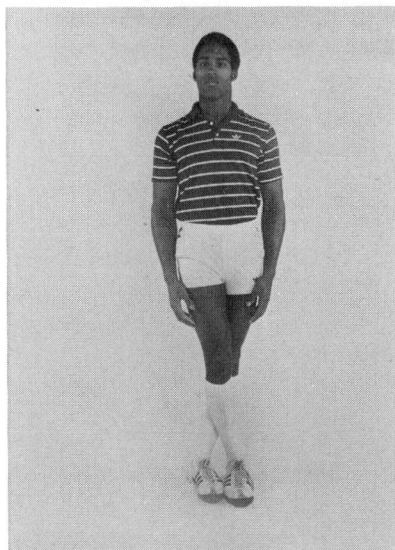

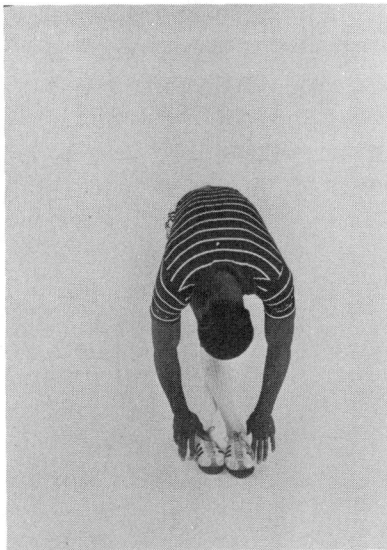

A good way to stretch the calves is to cross your legs and bend over. Try to touch your hands to your toes.

several inches to the right or left of your instep when bending down.

**Special considerations**: Since this is a rigorous stretching exercise it is important not to rush the movement or bounce at the bottom of the stretch.

### Jogging/Jumping Rope/Stationary Bike

**Basic movement**: The warm-up period should always be followed by about five minutes of easy cardiovascular exercise. You may elect to jog, either in place or on a measured course at a leisurely pace (about 10 minutes per mile). If you do not have facilities for jogging, rope jumping or stationary exercise bike work will suffice.

**What it does**: You should have loose muscles at the conclusion of the warm-up program. A light sweat and pulse rate of about 120-130 beats per minute indicates you are warmed up. This figure is about two-thirds of minimum heartbeat. To determine your theoretical maximum heart rate subtract your age from 220. To gain cardiovascular fitness, you need to keep your pulse rate above 120-130 beats for about thirty minutes, three times per week. All of the programs outlined here are designed to meet or exceed this goal. In this manner, the gym workout becomes an excellent cardiovascular conditioning program. The end of the warm-up period will accelerate your heart rate to this training level, and ease you into progressive resistance training.

**Variation on a theme**: Try to vary the rate of speed when jogging, jumping rope, or riding the exercise bike. By varying your level of exertion during this five-minute aerobic workout, the training benefits are enhanced.

**Special considerations**: Don't be concerned with speed or with showing how fit you are, especially if you are already a runner. That's not the purpose of this phase of the warmup. If you are already in good shape, you may find that you must increase the intensity of your jogging or rope jumping pace in order to get your heart rate up to training levels.

## THE FREEHAND EXERCISE PROGRAM

If you have never worked out with weights or if your last gym workout was more than a year or so ago, you should spend some time in the *freehand exercise program*. The freehand program is so-called because it does not require the use of weights or other gym apparatus, just some common household items. Freehand exercises are not "sissy work." They are used by most top strength training athletes as integral parts of their overall program. These exercises can be used later in your training as well, for a change of pace or when traveling.

Freehand exercises are important for the novice gym athlete because they have a tonic effect on the major muscles of the body. These exercises will give you the feeling, perhaps for the first time, of having a "pump" in your muscles. The pump, a term borrowed from bodybuilding, is the feeling you experience when heavy exercise causes blood to rush into and engorge a given muscle or groups of muscles. Your skin feels tight and you feel as though you could lift a car. The pump lets you know that you have worked a muscle hard enough for a training effect to occur.

The beginning freehand program is not a series of calisthenics, but a program that uses your own body weight as resistance. If you weigh 150 pounds, for example, you can use this weight as resistance in the same way you would use the plates on a barbell. The freehand program will consist of the following exercises: 1) Pushups,  2) Dips between chairs, 3) Rowing between chairs, 4)

Bent-leg sit-ups, 5) Bent-leg raises, 6) Bent-over twists, 7) Squats/ Lunges, 8) Calf raises, 9) Pullups. Unlike the warm-up exercises, it is impossible to say how many repetitions of each of these exercises you should begin with. Each person has differing strength levels and stamina. You will have to experiment to determine a proper starting place. As in all exercise programs, it pays to start off doing a little bit less than you think you can and gradually increasing your workload.

Whatever the number of repetitions you are able to do in the freehand program, you should always do at least two sets per exercise. You will benefit more by doing two sets of five repetitions each in the pushup than doing a single set of ten pushups. You should quickly work your way up to three sets of each exercise. When you can do three complete sets of each exercise, with minimal rest between sets, you are ready to proceed to weight work in the gym.

A complete three-set freehand program, including warm-up activities, should be completed in about forty-five minutes, and at most one hour. Rest periods should be no more than a minute between sets, and ideally only about thirty to forty-five seconds. Why is pace so important? You are attempting to build not only muscle strength and stamina, but also cardiovascular fitness. You must try keeping the activity level high enough during the workout so that your pulse rate is always about 130 beats a minute. Prolonged rest periods will interfere with cardiovascular development in the freehand program or any gym program for that matter.

Do enough repetitions so that the last few in the set require a concerted effort to complete while maintaining proper form. These last few reps are the ones that force the body to adapt to a higher fitness level, so they must be tough. Do not, however, get into any "macho" games by trying to do more than your body can handle. There is a fine line between maximum training capability and overtraining.

Keeping proper form during all exercises cannot be overemphasized. It is better to do five perfect pushups than ten sloppy ones. You can only cheat yourself by having sloppy form. The number of exercises you can do is unimportant.

Three workouts per week, spaced at least one day apart will give you the optimal results on the freehand program. Do not attempt to speed up your progress by working out more than three times per week, because the recuperation period between work-outs is as important as the workouts themselves.

An accomplished athlete need only stay on the freehand program for about two weeks before moving on to gymwork. A person who has spent several years or even decades getting out of shape should devote extra time to the freehand program. Generally, give yourself about one month to get into reasonable shape for every year that you spent out of shape. Otherwise, listen to your body and monitor your feelings. They will tell you when it is time to move on to harder work. When three sets of each exercise get too easy, you will know you can safely move on. You might find, especially if you have already joined a gym or health club, that you will want to phase into a complete gym program while you are still doing some of the freehand exercises. This is a good approach, because many of the freehand exercises will be encountered again in all the gym training programs, no matter how advanced your level.

## FREEHAND EXERCISES

### Pushups

**Basic movement:** Pushups are so basic to upper body development that they are often included in warm-up activities for advanced weight-training athletes. Place your hands on the floor approximately shoulder-width apart, as you lie face down. Exhale as you push yourself straight up off the floor until your arms are fully extended. Pause at the point of full arm extension and then slowly lower yourself (inhaling as you go down) until your chest touches the floor. Pause and repeat. If you are female, you may want to start out supporting the weight of your lower body on your knees, rather than your feet.

**What it does:** Pushups work the pectoral muscles of your chest, as well as the deltoid muscles of your shoulders and the triceps muscles of the back of your arms. You will feel a "pump" in all of these muscle groups if you do the pushup correctly.

**Variations on a theme:** By varying the placement of your hands, you emphasize the use of specific muscles in this exercise. For example, by positioning your hands more than shoulder-width apart you will put more strain on your chest muscles. Conversely, placing your hands only a foot apart affects your triceps muscles and your deltoids.

## Pushups

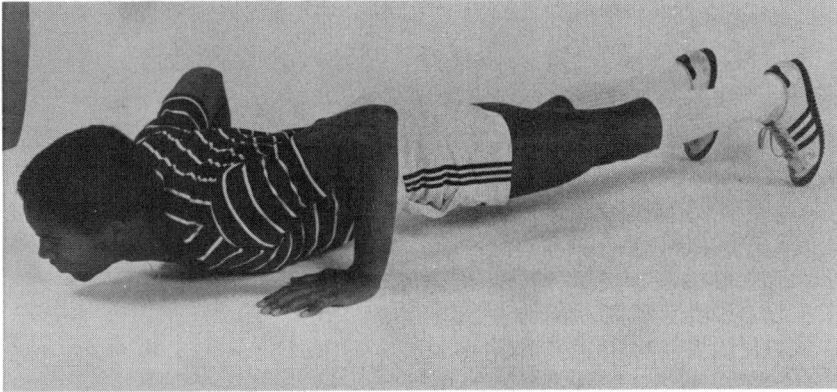

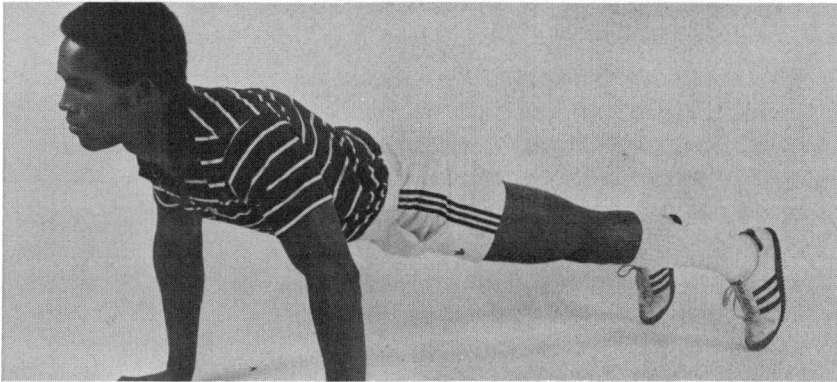

Pushups work the pectoral muscles of your chest and the deltoid muscles of your shoulders. Varying the placement of your hands will work different muscles.

**Special considerations:** Most people do pushups incorrectly. Make sure to keep the body straight throughout the movement. The movement should be fluid and each rep should take at least three seconds to complete. Try to work up to three sets of twenty repetitions each.

### Chair Dips

**Basic movement:** Place two chairs that are sturdy enough to support your weight shoulder-width apart with the backs facing each other. Stand between the chairs and place one hand on each of the chair backs. Lift your feet slightly so that you are supporting your body weight with your arms. Then lower yourself until your shoulders are about level with the tops of the chairs. Pause at the bottom of the movement and raise yourself using your arm, shoulder and chest muscles until your arms are fully extended again.

**What it does**: This is an excellent exercise for the triceps, deltoids, and the pectoral muscles of the chest. You should feel "pumped" in all of these muscle groups after doing a set of dips.

**Variations on a theme**: When you do dips in an upright position, you will find that you feel the effort more in the back of your arms and in your shoulders. If you lean forward slightly, your chest muscles, particularly the pectorals, get more exercise. A good plan is to alternate these variations in your workout.

**Special considerations**: Dips are tough exercises. You may only be able to do one or two reps at a time at the beginning. Nonetheless, try to do three sets of dips in each workout, even if each set includes only one rep. Proper form is important in this exercise, if only to prevent injury. Do the movement slowly, taking at least three seconds per repetition. The effect of controlling your body weight as you lower yourself is every bit as important as the upward movement. You will experience this in almost every exercise. If you lower yourself rapidly, allowing inertia to take your body to the bottom of the movement, you are robbing yourself of half the training benefits of this or any other progressive resistance exercise. Using proper form, work up to twenty reps or more.

### Rowing Between Chairs

**Basic movement**: The first two exercises of the freehand program were concerned mainly with the development of the front of the upper body. You will now work the muscles of your back, especially the latissimus dorsi muscles of the side of your back and the spinal erector muscles on either side of your spine. Use the same two chairs as in the dips. Place the chairs back-to-back and about four feet apart and a broomstick across the tops of the chairs. Lie face up on the floor between the chairs and grip the broomstick with your hands placed about shoulder-width apart and your palms facing upward. Now pull your body upward, using your feet to anchor your lower body, until your chest touches the broomstick. Keeping your body perfectly straight, lower yourself again, inhaling on the way to the floor. Movement should only be in your arms.

**What it does**: By working the muscles of the back, you will prepare the body for a number of rowing exercises that will be introduced later. If you have lower back trouble, this exercise strengthens muscles there.

**Variations on a theme**: By placing your hands on the broomstick so that your palms face toward you, this exercise will also work your biceps muscles.

**Special considerations**: Rowing movements, like dips, can be tough in the beginning. Most find it especially uncomfortable to breathe while rowing. Make sure you exhale as you raise yourself to the bar and inhale on the way down. Work up to three sets of fifteen repetitions each and you will be on your way to strengthening your back. You may also want to use a weightlifting belt in this exercise, especially if you experience considerable soreness in the lower back from doing this movement.

### Bent-Leg Sit-Ups

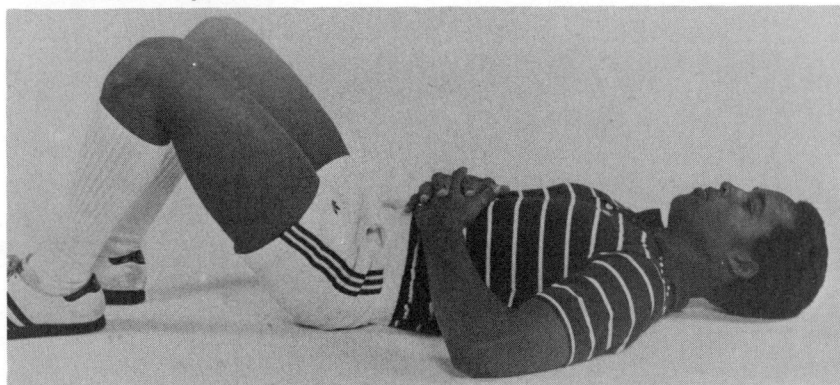

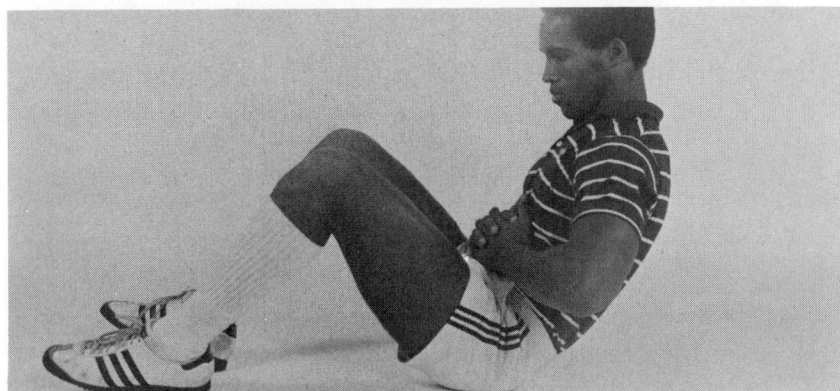

**Basic movement**: Place your feet under a heavy piece of furniture and lie down on your back so that your legs are bent at your

**Bent-Leg Sit-Ups**

Bending the knees in a sit-up concentrates the exercise to the abdominals.

knees at about a 45-degree angle. Hold your hands over your abdomen with your fingers interlocked. Now raise your trunk, stopping when you are about three-quarters of the way up. Lower your body, stopping about three-quarters of the way down. Breathe in on the way down and exhale on the way up.

**What it does**: Bent-knee sit-ups are one of those basic exercises that can't be ignored. Bending the knees concentrates the exercise on the abdominal muscles, especially the upper abdominals, and reduces the use of the hip flexors. In addition, bending the legs at the knee reduces the strain on the lower back muscles.

**Variations on a theme**: Twist your body from left to right on both the upward and downward movements.

**Special considerations**: Refrain from going all the way up and all the way down because this variation keeps continuous tension on the abdominals. Do not hurry the repetitions; try for a smooth, fluid movement. Doing sit-ups faster will not take off fat quicker. Work up to three sets of twenty-five repetitions each and you will

### Bent-Leg Sit-Ups

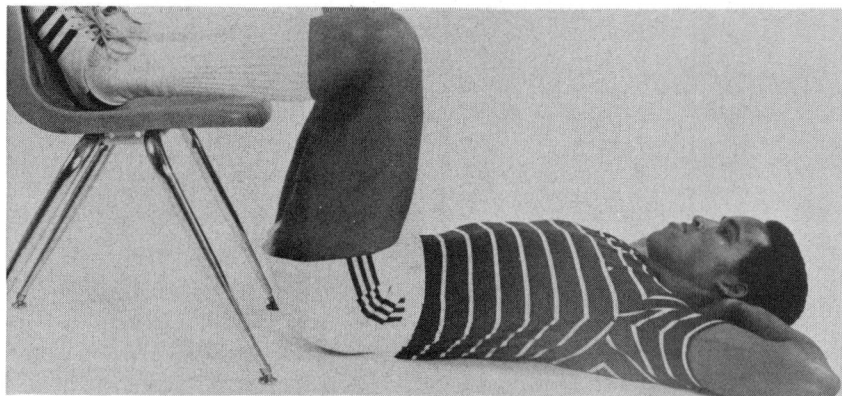

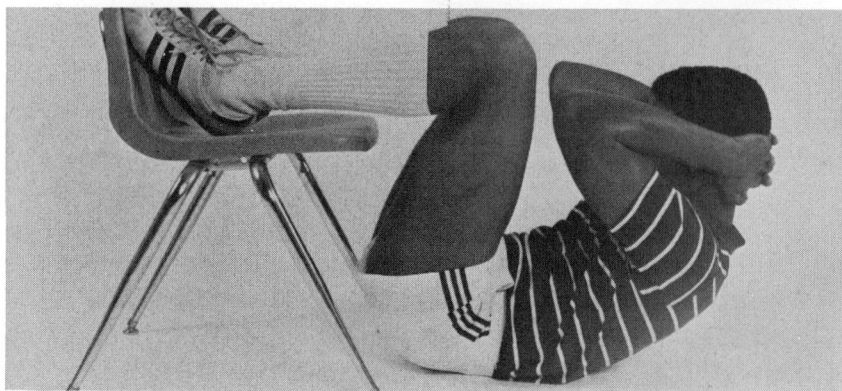

Sit-ups using a chair to prop up your legs are the most difficult variation.

soon notice a difference in muscle tone and the size of your waist. It is virtually impossible to increase the size of the waistline by doing abdominal exercises.

### Bent-Leg Raises

**Basic movement**: Lie on your back with your hands under your buttocks and your legs straight out. Keeping your chin on your chest, bring your knees up to your chest. Inhale as you lower your legs again, making sure that you keep your feet off the ground as your legs are fully extended.

**What it does**: This movement develops the muscles of the lower abdomen and the hip flexors of the front of the thighs.

**Variations on a theme**: Hold the extended leg position for a few seconds to maximize tension on the lower abdominals.

**Special considerations**: As in the sit-up, resistance is not as important as repetitions. Work up to three sets of twenty repetitions.

### Bent-Leg Raises

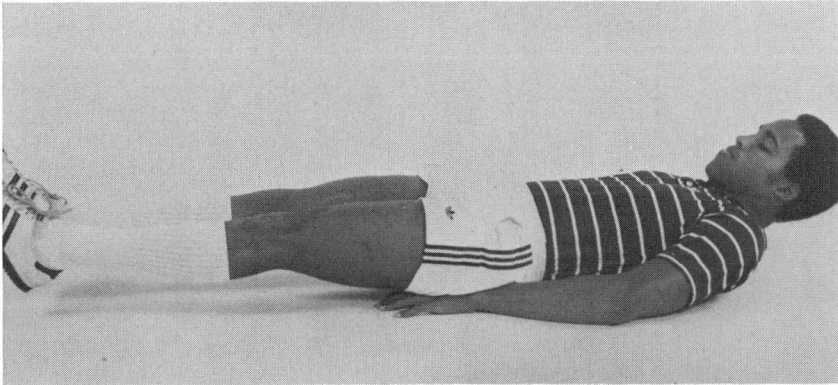

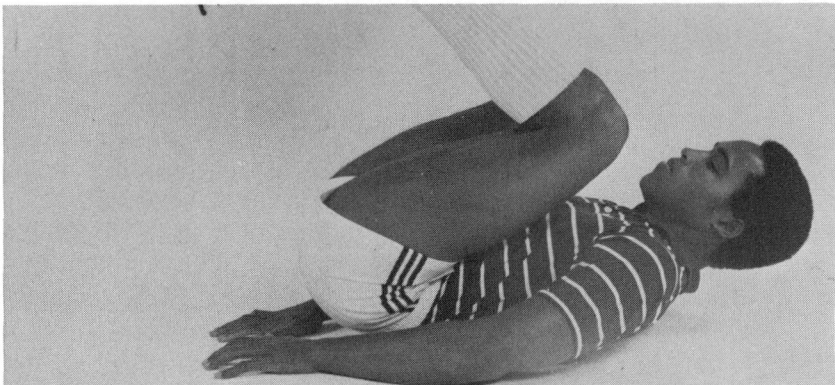

Bent-leg raises develop muscles of the lower abdomen and the hip flexors.

## Bent-Over Twists

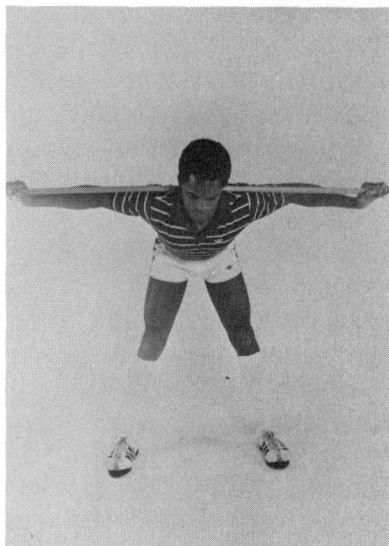

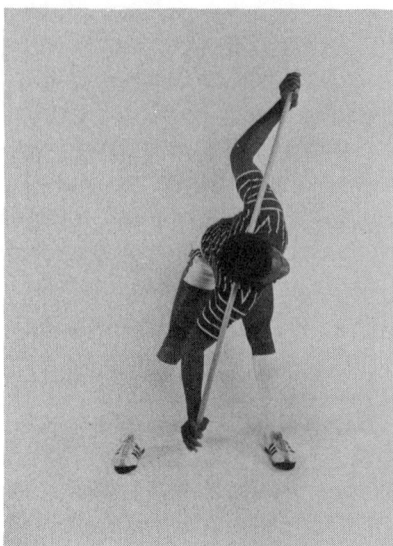

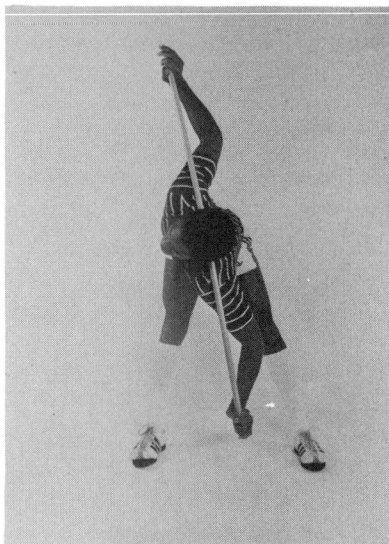

Use a broom or pole for the bent-over twists, alternating the movement between the feet. This works the oblique muscles of the waist.

## Bent-Over Twists

**Basic movement**: Place a broomstick behind your neck, grasping it with a wide grip. Hold your legs stiff while standing, and keep your feet about shoulder-width apart. Bend forward until your upper body is parallel with the floor. Now twist your body in half-circle motions, bringing the ends of the broomstick down to touch your insteps, alternating right to left.

**What it does**: Twists work the oblique muscles at the sides of the waist. They also loosen the muscles of the abdomen and lower back. Combined with the other abdominal exercises, they work the abdominals from a number of different angles.

**Variations on a theme**: Start the twists from an erect position.

**Special considerations**: Strive for high repetition sets, using rapid, full-twisting motions. Try to do three sets of fifty twists, with one right/left series counting as one rep.

## Squats/Lunges

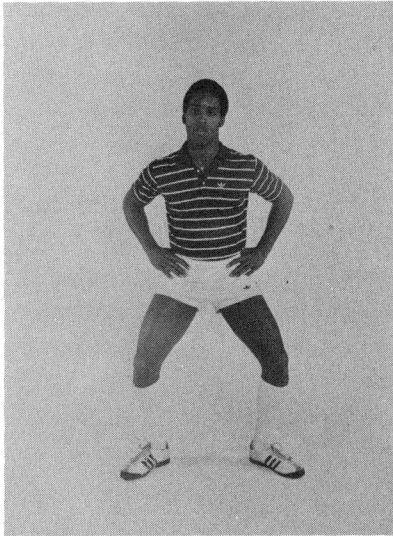

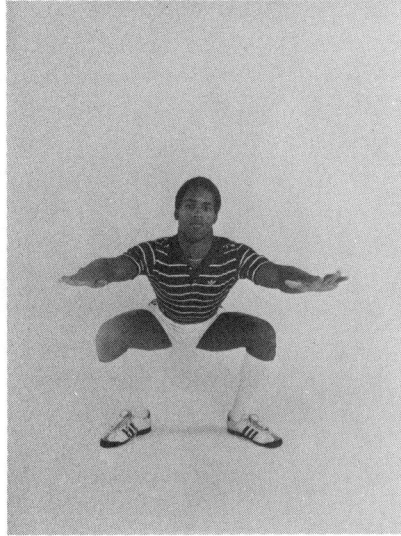

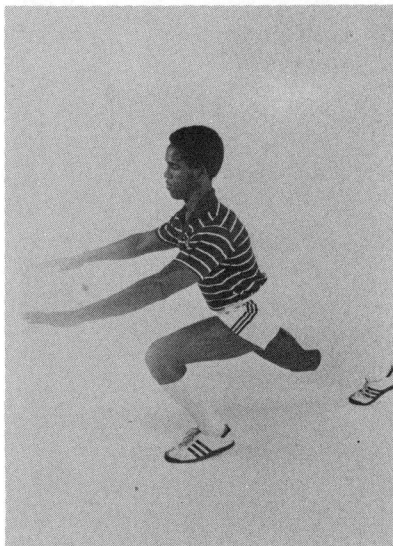

The lunge requires balance as well as strength. In the squat, both legs should be bent until parallel with the floor. Both exercises build and define the entire thigh.

### Squats/Lunges

**Basic movement**: Stand with your feet about one foot apart and your hands on your hips. To perform the squat, bend at your knees and lower yourself until your legs are parallel with the floor. Extend your arms in front of you for balance as you squat. Keeping your back straight, return to the starting position. The lunge is also performed from the standing position. Lunge forward with one leg, allowing that leg to bend at almost a 45-degree angle while keeping your trailing leg straight. Then, pushing with your forward leg, lift yourself back to the standing position. Alternate legs and repeat.

**What it does**: Both the squat and the lunge will build and define the entire thigh, especially the muscles of the front thigh. The lunge is slightly better at separating the muscle groups of the thigh from one another. In the freehand program, these two movements can be done interchangeably. Both exercises will also firm and strengthen the buttocks muscles.

**Variations on a theme**: These exercises involve large muscle groups in the body. Hence, if done with vigor they provide cardio-vascular training effects.

**Special considerations**: Proper form is especially important in doing squats and lunges. You will eventually be doing these exercises with weights and there is a good possibility of injury if bad habits creep in now. Do not lower yourself all the way during the squat; this stresses your knee joints unnecessarily. Keep your back straight at all times to prevent lower back strain. A weightlifting belt is an important safety feature in this exercise. Breathe in as you lower yourself and exhale on the upward movement.

### Calf Raises

**Basic movement**: Calf raises can be done with your toes resting on a book and your heels resting on the floor. Using a chair for balance, raise yourself up and down in a rhythmic fashion by pushing off with your feet.

**What it does**: Calf raises develop both the gastrocnemius and soleus muscles of the calf, as well as increasing flexibility in the Achilles tendon.

**Variations on a theme**: After you have done this movement for a while you can do calf raises using only one leg at a time.

**Special considerations**: The calf is comprised of dense muscle

## Calf Raises

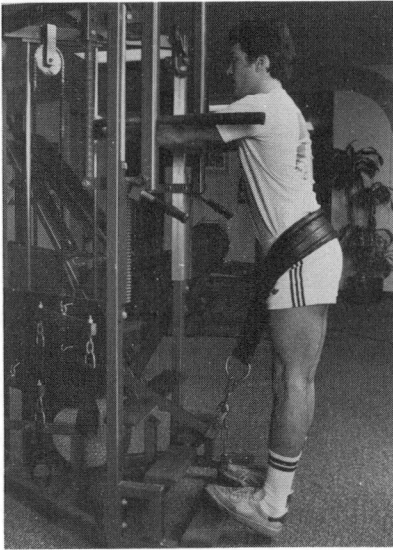

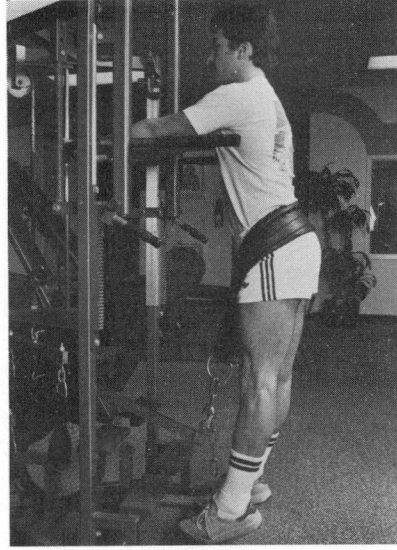

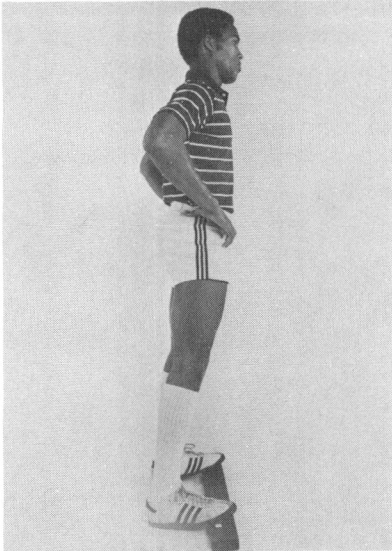

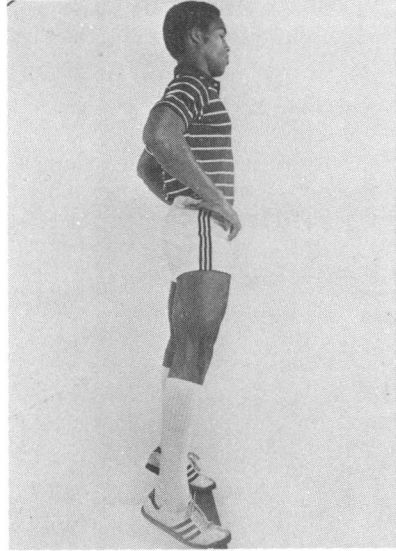

Calf raises can be done using a harness on some Nautilus machines. A harness concentrates the action to the calf muscles. You don't need a Nautilus to do calf raises. A wood board is all it takes.

fibers, which are difficult to develop without cramping. Do the movement slowly and completely; later you will be doing similar exercises with weights added as resistance.

## Pullups

**Basic movement**: Grip the chinning bar with your hands at shoulder width and your palms facing away from you. Raise yourself until your chin is even with the bar. Inhale as you lower yourself back to the fully extended starting position.

**What it does**: Pullups are another basic exercise. They build and define the entire upper body, especially the shoulders and back. You will notice a pump in the chest and arm muscles.

**Variations on a theme**: Variations abound with pullups. If you grip the bar with your palms facing toward you, you will work your biceps more. The wider your grip on the bar, the more difficult the exercise becomes and the more the work is directed to your lats. You can also pull yourself up so that your neck is drawn under the bar instead of chinning the bar. This variation is best done with your palms facing forward, and develops your back, especially the trapezius muscles of your upper back, to a remarkable degree. Pullups are difficult, particularly at the end of the workout. Do not use your feet or legs to hold yourself up and don't swing yourself back and forth to gain upward momentum. Work up to three sets of eight to ten reps each. Make sure you breathe in on the way down and exhale as you raise yourself.

**Pullups**

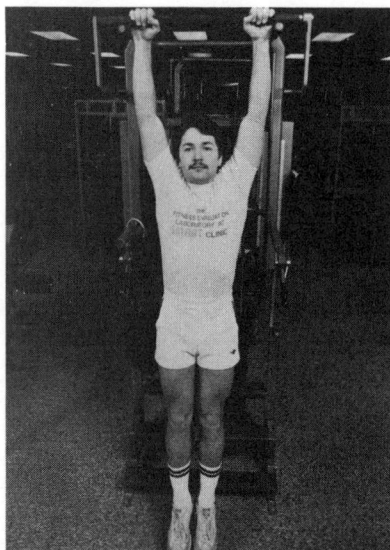

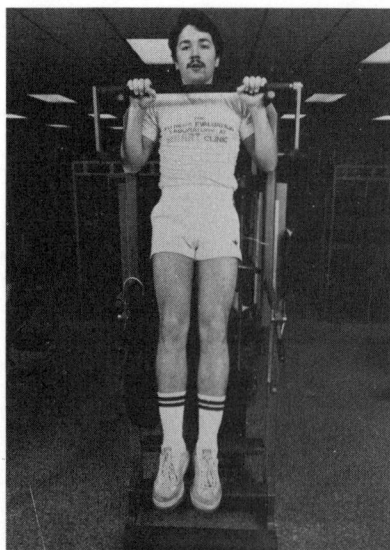

Pullups call for the palms of the hands to be facing away from you. Be sure you get full extension with the arms.

## WARMDOWN

The warmdown is as important as the warmup. Because muscular force is a function of both the contraction of a muscle and the *range* of contraction, stretching after contraction is important for maintaining flexibility and power. Many weight training athletes work very hard in the contractile portion of their programs and then neglect the post-workout warmdown. Their muscles actually tend to shorten and this leads to the musclebound look; the muscles always appear to be flexed. In a comprehensive training program you don't want this to happen. Test yourself periodically to make sure that you are developing properly. Measure the circumference of your upper arm when it is relaxed and when it is fully contracted. During contraction your arm should be about 10 percent larger than when relaxed. The increased circumference results from a muscle that can contract over a wide range of motion.

To warm down after the workout, follow the same exercises used to warm up. Follow the stretching exercises with jogging, swimming, rope jumping, or bicycling. These aerobic activities can also be conducted on non-workout days. Just be certain that you don't do too much if you are a beginner. Persistent fatigue is an indication of overtraining.

Aerobic activities are an important part of the comprehensive freehand program. Twenty minutes of aerobic work three times a week will not only develop cardiovascular fitness, but also stretch the long skeletal muscles and burn large amounts of energy. The complete freehand program, including warmup, progressive resistance exercises, and ten minutes of warmdown will burn between 500 and 700 calories, depending on the intensity of work and your present body mass.

## FREEHAND PROGRAM HINTS

Restricting yourself to three workouts per week will allow the greatest fitness gains and guard against overtraining. Refer often to your self-evaluation and training logs. Add more reps only when you feel able to do so. After the workout, pose in the mirror and view the body from all angles. Note your progress and parts of the body that need more work. You will soon begin to see muscle definition where none previously existed.

When the freehand program no longer seems a challenge move on to the weight training program. You should be doing three sets of each freehand exercise and the indicated number of repetitions. If you were really out of shape when you started the freehand program, it may take you one, two, even three months to work up to this fitness level. Don't let this concern you, however. Work at your own pace.

# 5

# The Basic Gym
# Training Program

This basic training program is designed to use apparatus, found in gyms and health clubs, which optimizes strength and endurance. Later, as an intermediate gym trainee, your body should look fit and athletic and you may then individualize your training and branch off onto any tangent you desire. But no matter what direction you choose, you will continue to use these basic gym exercises throughout your gym training. That's because basic movements develop the large muscle groups, which include:

1) Chest—pectorals,
2) Back—latissimus dorsi and spinal erectors,
3) Shoulders—deltoids,
4) Arms—biceps and triceps,
5) Abdominals—rectus abdominus and obliques,
6) Legs—quadriceps and hamstrings,
7) Calves—gastrocnemius.

Later in your gym training you will be introduced to more complicated exercises that work specific muscles. For detail work to be successful you must have the proper foundation. The basic movements also allow you to concentrate on maximum effort and proper form.

The program you follow in the basic training program will be determined by the types of equipment found in your gym or home. If your gym has free-weight equipment and Nautilus or Universal machines, you can do the basic exercises on these apparatus. Each exercise in this and succeeding sections will be presented for the free weight, Universal Gym, and Nautilus machine.

Based on your training in the freehand program, you should

know how much work you can handle in one workout. Use this knowledge to choose a proper starting weight. A rule of thumb is that the weight should be light enough so that you do three sets of eight to ten repetitions in every movement. It must be heavy enough, however, so that the last two or three reps in each set are difficult to complete in proper form. Remember that exercise strain is cumulative—the last few exercises will be much tougher than the preceding ones, and you will have to choose your weights accordingly. The eight-to-ten repetitions per set is not an arbitrary number. It represents the optimum compromise between high rep/low resistance sets, which develop definition, and high resistance/low rep sets, which are more effective at developing power. Later you may tailor your workouts to accommodate these training variations.

The basic program should be completed between forty-five minutes and an hour. Maintain a steady pace, resting no more than thirty to forty-five seconds between sets. The following notation will be used for describing a workout: 110/3 X 10 (sample) is short for three sets of ten reps each using 110 lb. of weight. You may use this system in your personal training log.

## THE BASIC PROGRAM

In the basic program, you will do a variation of the following routine:

1) Warm-up exercises (as in the freehand program)

2) Chest exercises (bench press)

3) Back exercises (bent rowing, lat pulldowns, pullovers, deadlifts)

4) Shoulder exercises (military press, seated press, dumbbell press)

5) Upper arm exercises (upright curls, reverse curls, triceps extensions)

6) Abdominal exercises (bent-leg raises, sit-ups, knee pull-ups)

7) Leg exercises (squats/lunges, leg extensions/curls, calf raises)

8) Supplementary exercises (dips, chinning)

9) Warm-down exercises (as in the freehand program)

Variations of each exercise will allow you a great deal of freedom, even within the basic program. These variations can be used later with your individualized exercises and techniques, to tailor your gym program to your needs and goals. There are hundreds of exercises that could comprise a good basic program and authors disagree on which to include in a basic program. Several variations on the basic movements will be presented here. Not every basic program will include all of these variations or exercises, nor should they. Gym training regimens are not straightjackets, but simply guides to progress. You are responsible for choosing the movements that seem to benefit you the most. For example, while the bench press is generally considered the top basic exercise for the development of the chest, people with especially long arms sometimes find that this movement fatigues their arms long before their chest muscles get sufficient work.

## NOTES ON USING FREE WEIGHTS, UNIVERSAL GYMS, AND NAUTILUS MACHINES

In most cases you will be able to pull or push the barbell or dumbbell into the correct starting position denoted in each exercise. Always lift free weights using the strength of your legs and hips, keeping the back straight. If you need help, enlist the aid of your training partner or one of the gym personnel. Never attempt to show off and lift or move a weight that might be beyond your capacity.

Most gyms have racks in which free weights are stored. When you are done using a weight, put it back in the rack you took it from. A gym cluttered with loose weights is dangerous.

Nautilus machines have directions written on them on how to adjust the seating. Check for proper adjustment as follows: your shoulder should be slightly below the elbow during the contraction phase; elbows must be lined up so that they move along the axis of the cam. If any of the pads roll over your arm or leg as you move, the seat is not adjusted correctly.

Some Nautilus machines have foot pedals to take resistance off working muscles. These include some arm machines, the pullover machine, the chest machine, and others. In machines with pedals, seat yourself, fasten the lap belt (if there is one), and press down on the pedal enough to slip your arms into the working parts of the machine. When you let go of the pedal, you can then perform the necessary repetitions. When you are done with the machine, reverse the procedure you followed to get into it and step free from the machine. On non-pedal machines, you just slide your arms free and walk away.

The Universal Gym is easy to use. Put the pin holding the weight stack under the proper number of plates and you can then perform the exercise. It is a good idea to visually check the pulleys and pin placement to be sure they are in place.

Gymwork should be conducted with safety in mind. The potential for injury always exists when using heavy weights or machines. If something looks defective, don't use it; alert the gym personnel. Before you use any weight, make sure the collars or fasteners are secure.

## BASIC PROGRAM EXERCISES

### CHEST EXERCISES
**Bench Press**

**Basic movement:**

**Free weight**: Lie on a flat bench with your head at one end of the bench and your feet flat on the floor. Take a shoulder-width grip on the barbell, palms facing forward and perpendicular to the floor. Raise the bar off the upright holder, bend your elbows, and let the bar descend to your chest at nipple level. Push the bar back to the starting position by straightening your arms.

**Universal Gym**: Lie on the flat bench (head pointed toward the weights) at the bench press station. Raise and lower the handles connected to the weight stack using the same motion as for free weights.

**Nautilus**: Seat yourself in the Nautilus chest machine and lean back on the seat, which is at a 45-degree angle. Place your feet on the pedals and grasp the pressing handles with your palms facing each other. With an assisting push from your feet on the pedals, force the handles away from your body until your arms are fully extended.

**What it does**: The bench press develops the chest; it also trains the muscles of the shoulder and the triceps muscles of the back of the arm.

**Variations on a theme**: Using free weights, and to some extent the Universal Gym, hand position can be varied. A wide grip

## Bench Press

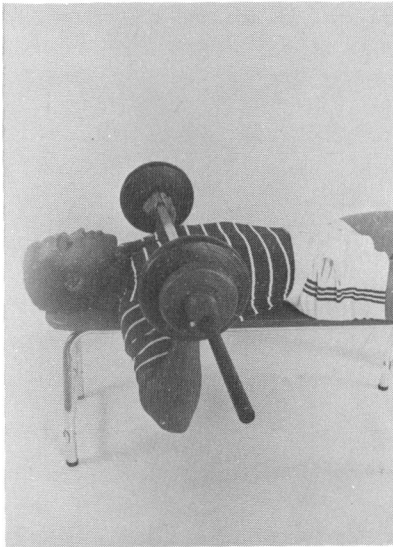

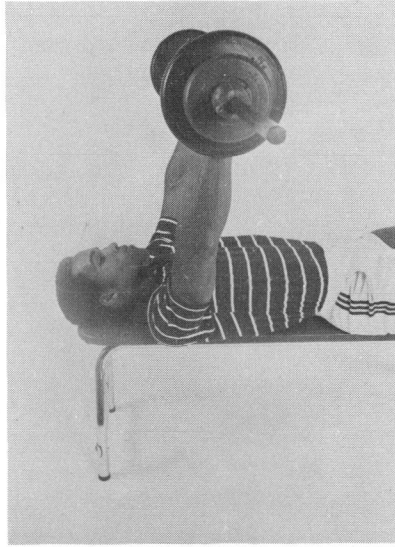

Begin the bench press with the bar at your chin. Push the bar up until your arms are fully extended.

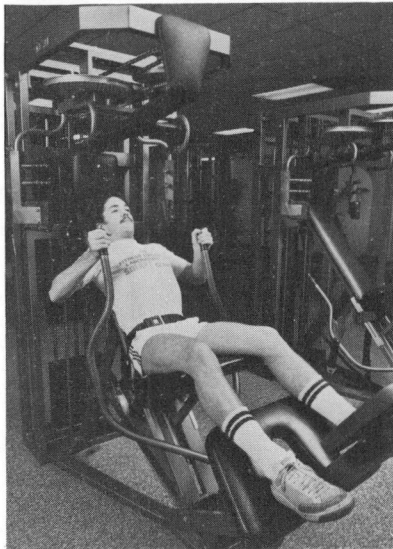

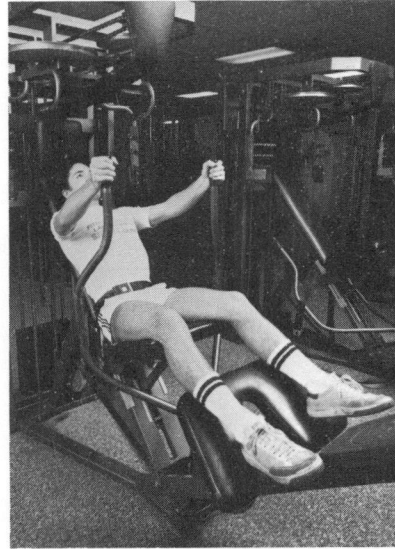

A Nautilus chest machine looks like the cockpit of some alien space ship. The action is similar to the free weight bench press.

stresses the outer pectoral muscles while a close grip, with the hands a foot or so apart, forces more effort from the muscles in the lower and central part of the chest and the triceps. Make sure to inhale on the downward movement and exhale as the weight is raised. Lower the weight slowly and completely, counteracting the force of gravity at all times.

## BACK EXERCISES
### Bent Rowing

**Basic movement**: Place a barbell in front of you on the floor. Stand so that your feet are about shoulder-width apart. Bend down at your waist and grasp the bar with your palms downward and your hands placed about one foot apart. In this bent-over position, raise the bar to your upper abdomen and then lower the bar until your arms are fully extended, bending only your elbows.

**What it does**: Rowing develops the lats, the spinal erectors, and the muscles of the lower back. As in all push/pull exercises, a pump in the arms should be noticed when doing this movement.

**Variations on a theme**: Gripping the bar with the hands placed about six inches apart concentrates the effort directly on the lats.

**Special considerations**: As with all rowing motions, breathing is difficult. Inhale as the weight is lowered and exhale as the weight is brought up to the upper abdomen. Make sure to bring the weight up until it touches the upper abdomen and concentrate on moving only the elbows, so that the back muscles do most of the work.

**Bent Rowing**

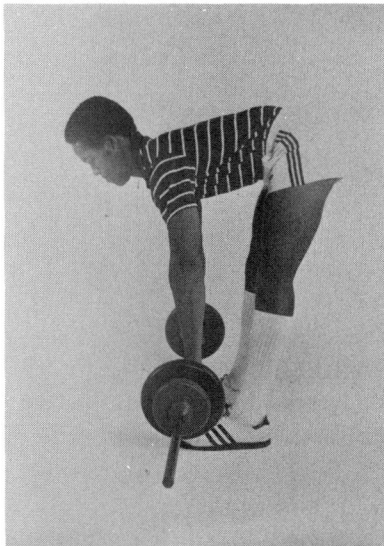

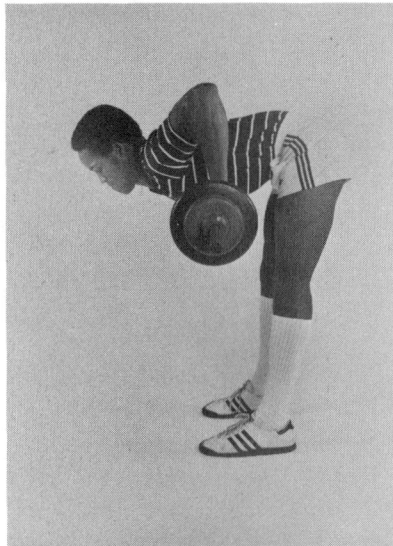

Exhale as the weight is brought up to the upper abdomen in the bent rowing free weight exercise.

**Lat Pulldowns**

**Basic movement**: At the lat pulldown station of the Universal Gym or at the specialized lat pulldown apparatus, grasp the handles at the ends of the bar so that your hands are six to twelve inches more than shoulder-width apart and your palms are facing forward. Sit or kneel in front of the machine, facing the weight stack. Pull the bar down until it touches the base of your neck behind your head. Return to the starting position, arms straight, and pull the next rep to the front of your neck. Alternate each rep front to back for the full set.

**What it does**: Pulldowns are the primary exercise for the latissimus dorsi, with secondary emphasis on the deltoids, biceps, and forearms. These muscles are used for pushing and pulling.

**Variations on a theme**: Pulldowns can also be done using a close grip, with your palms facing toward you. In this variation, the bar is pulled down toward your chest. You will work different muscles doing pulldowns in this fashion.

**Special considerations**: The latissimus muscle pulls the upper arms down and back, so emphasize pulling your elbows down and back on each rep. Be sure to let the weight up gradually as you raise your arms to the starting position.

**Pullovers**

**Basic movement**:

**Free weight**: Lie across a flat bench on your back so that your body is perpendicular to the long axis of the bench and your shoulders are directly on the bench. Keep your feet flat on the floor. Grip a dumbbell with both hands holding one of the ends. As you raise it in front of you, it should be aligned straight up and down. Extend your outstretched arms behind your head and lower the dumbbell until it touches the floor. Then raise the dumbbell, keeping your arms stiff, until it is suspended directly above your chest.

**Nautilus**: Enter the Nautilus pullover machine and adjust the seat so that your shoulders are about even with the Nautilus cam. Push down on the pedals until you can put your elbows on the large pads attached to the movement arm. Rest the outer part of your arms against the outer angled pads on each side. Grasp the bar behind your neck and let go of the pedals with your feet. Allow your elbows to travel as far behind your head as possible.

## Pullovers

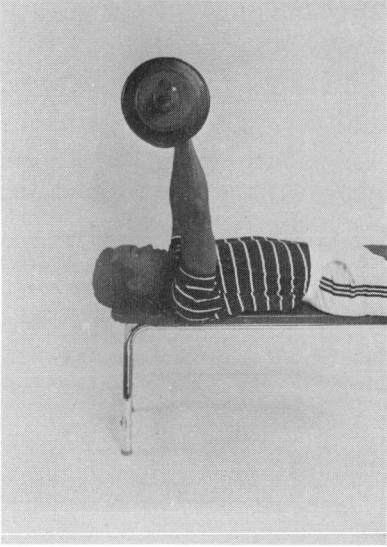

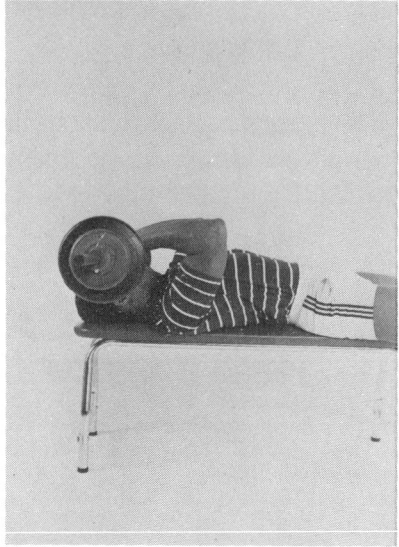

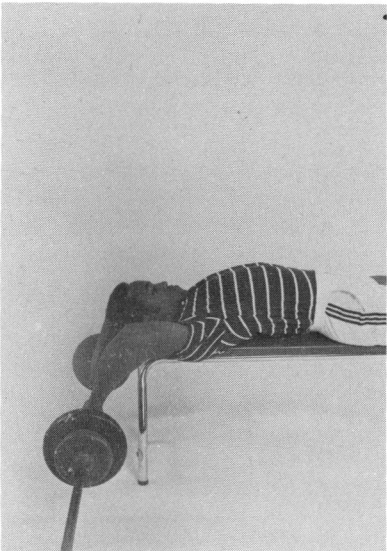

Pullovers can be done with a barbell or a dumbbell. Start with the weight over your chest and lower it behind your head while lying on a bench. Don't use too much weight.

## Pullovers (Cont.)

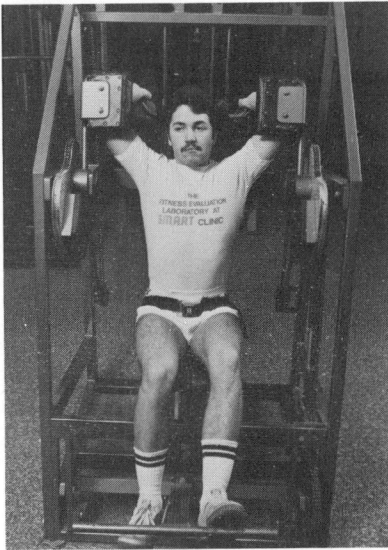

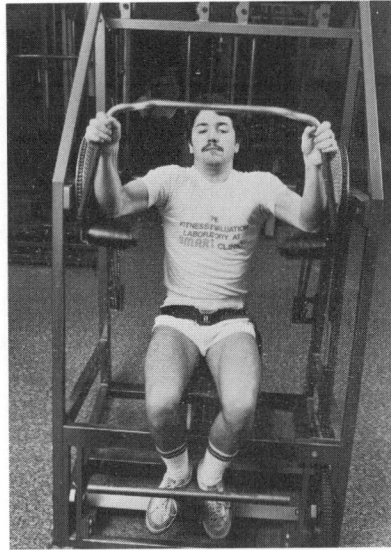

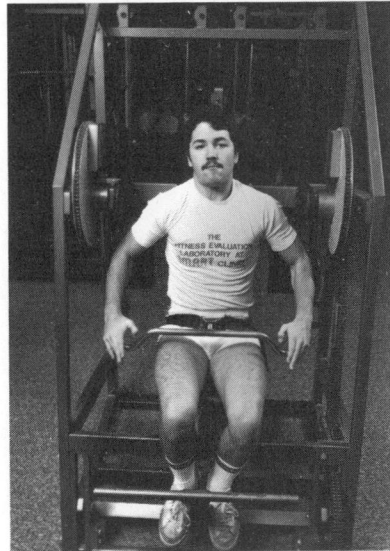

Adjust the Nautilus pullover machine so that your shoulders are about even with the Nautilus cam. This exercise works the rib cage.

Then push the pads in a semicircle with your elbows going as far down and as far forward as they can. The movement bar will usually be resting across your abdomen. Return along the same arc to the starting position.

**What it does**: These stretching and pulling motions are different from those produced by the lat pulldown, and the exercises work to expand the rib cage.

**Variations on a theme**: Hold the position with your arms extended as far in back of your head as possible for a few seconds in the middle of a rep to achieve maximum stretch.

**Special considerations**: Many initially find pullovers very difficult. If you are working on the Nautilus machine and can't finish a rep, just press the foot pedal, which will remove the resistance and allow you to take your arms from the machine.

### Deadlifts

**Basic movement**: Stand up to a barbell with your shins resting against the bar. Keep your feet about shoulder-width apart and your toes pointed slightly outward. Bend down and grasp the bar with an overhand (palms facing toward your body) grip so that your hands are about two feet apart and your palms face your shins. Bend your legs until your upper thighs are parallel with the ground. Arch your back slightly to put tension on the spinal erector muscles of your lower back. Keep your head upright and facing forward throughout the exercise. Then pull the barbell up along your legs, first by straightening your legs and then by extending at your hips so that your body is once again upright. At this point the barbell will be resting across your thighs. Lower the barbell slowly along the same path.

**What it does**: This exercise strengthens the spinal erectors of the lower back and the muscles of the front thigh, with secondary emphasis on the upper back, the hamstrings, and the hip extensors. The muscles of the abdomen and calf act as stabilizers. The deadlift develops lifting strength.

**Variations on a theme**: To work the trapezius muscles of the upper back, try shrugging your shoulders at the top of the movement.

**Special considerations**: It is vitally important that you keep the leg straightening/hip extension sequence as you lift the bar and the hip flexion/leg bending sequence as you lower the bar. Always keep the bar as close as possible to your body. Follow these pre-cautions to avoid lower back strain, and use a weightlifting belt as added protection.

## Deadlift

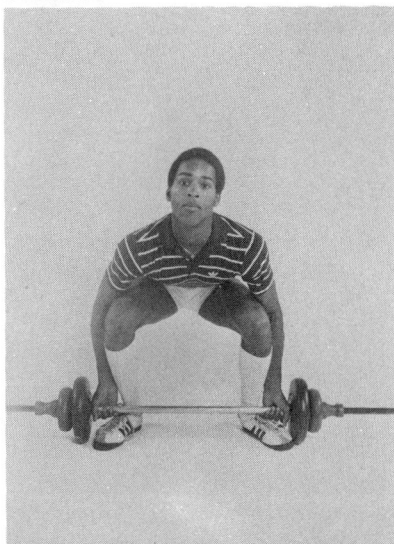

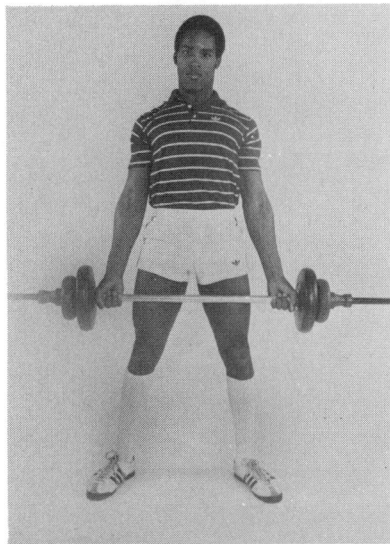

During the deadlift it is important that you keep the legs straight as you lift the bar and as you lower it. Keep the weight as close as possible to your body.

## SHOULDER EXERCISES
### Military Press

**Basic movement**: With your feet about shoulder-width apart and your toes pointed slightly outward, grasp a barbell that lies on the floor; use the overhand grip. Now stand erect with the barbell, first straightening your legs and then extending at your hips. Bring the bar up to your shoulders so that it rests across the front of them and at the base of your neck. Then push the bar straight up until your elbows are locked and the bar is directly over your head. Bend your elbows and return the bar to your shoulders. When you have performed the required number of reps, return the bar to the floor by bending first your legs and then flexing your hips.

**What it does**: The military press works the deltoid muscles of the shoulders and the triceps muscles of the backs of the arms. It also trains the upper pectorals and the trapezius. The lower back, abdominals, and legs act as stabilizers.

## Military Press

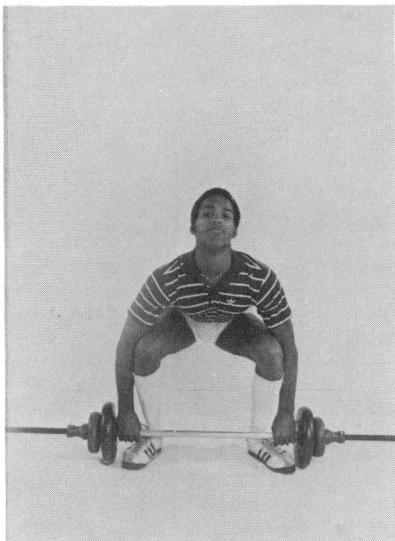

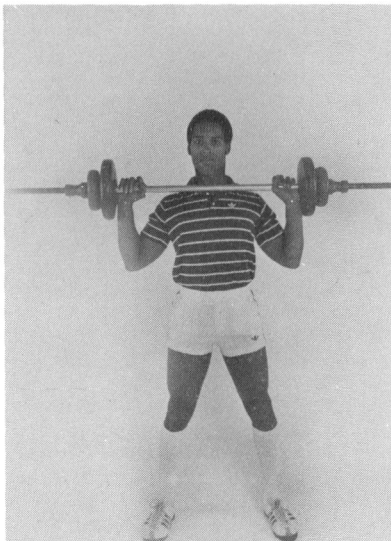

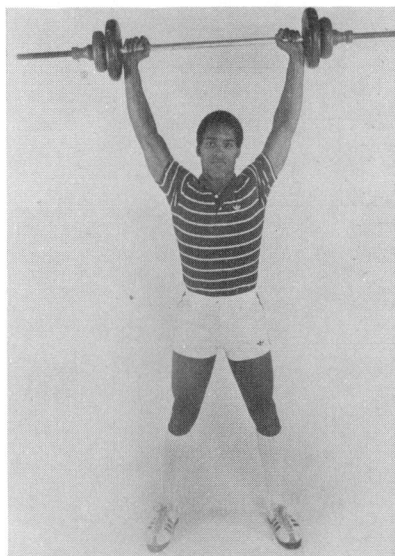

Bend down to grasp the barbell to begin the military press. A power surge brings the barbell to your shoulders and then push the weight over your head.

## Military Press (Cont.)

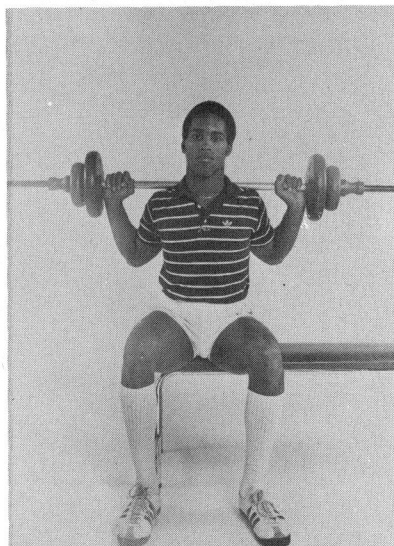

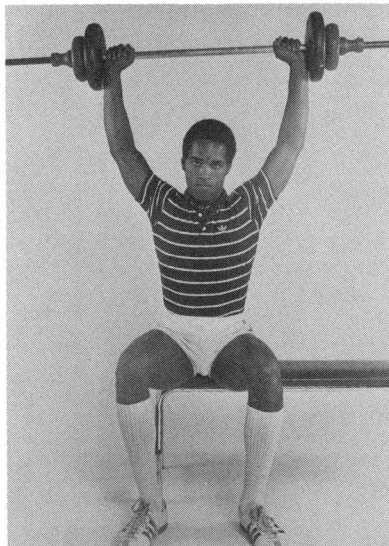

You can do the military press while seated. Remaining seated for the military press takes some strain off the back.

**Variations on a theme**: The military press can also be done from the seated position, which takes some strain off the back. The front deltoids can be exercised more specifically by raising the bar over the head and then lowering it behind rather than in front of the neck. You might want to alternate the front and back variations.

**Special considerations**: Minimize bending backward as you raise the bar. Bending makes the movement easier, but also causes undue strain on your lower back. Avoid hitting your nose with the bar as you press it upward. While this sounds silly, broken noses have resulted from this exercise.

### Seated Presses (Universal and Nautilus)

**Basic movement**:

**Universal Gym**: Sit on a bench in front of the Universal Gym pressing station handles, facing the machine and grasping the handles with an overhand grip. Your palms should be facing away from your body and your hands about shoulder-width apart. Push the handles straight up until your arms are fully extended and your elbows locked. Now bend your elbows, lower the handles to the starting position, and repeat.

**Nautilus machine**: Adjust the seat until you can grasp the handles exactly at shoulder height. Your palms should be facing one another and your back firmly against the back rest. Cross your ankles directly under your knees and fasten the seat belt, if one is available. Then push the handles until your elbows are locked. Bend your elbows and lower the bar to the starting position.

**What it does**: This motion works the same muscles as the military press, namely the deltoids, triceps, pectorals and trapezius.

**Variations on a theme**: The Universal Gym and Nautilus machine do not lend themselves to variations in these movements.

**Special considerations**: Try to keep your feet off the floor when doing presses while seated. Otherwise, your legs will unavoidably assist the pressing motion. Using your legs can mean as much as a 10 to 15 percent strength advantage in the military press.

**Seated Presses**

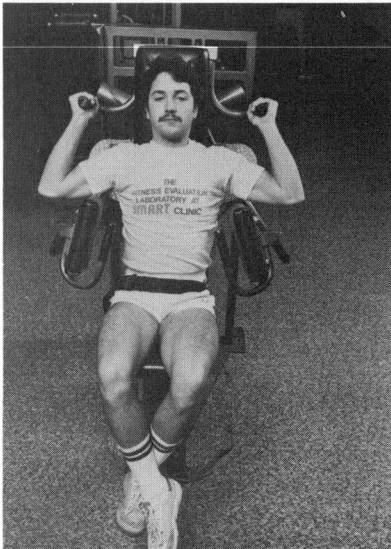

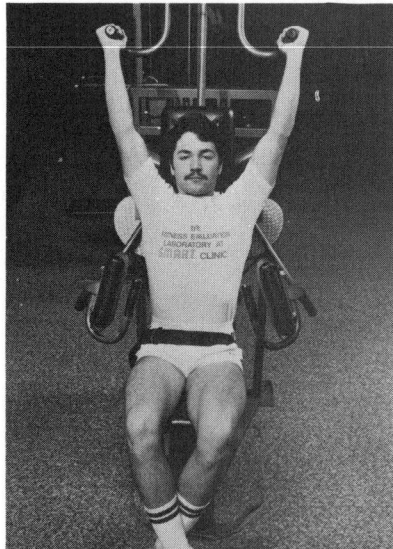

In the Nautilus military press machine push the handles up until your elbows are locked. Using the seat belt helps isolate the movement.

## Dumbbell Presses

**Basic movement**: Stand with your feet about shoulder-width apart and your toes pointed slightly outward. Grasp a dumbbell in each hand and bring them to shoulder height as if you were going to do the military press with a barbell. At your shoulders, your palms should be facing forward, similar to the position in

## Dumbbell Presses

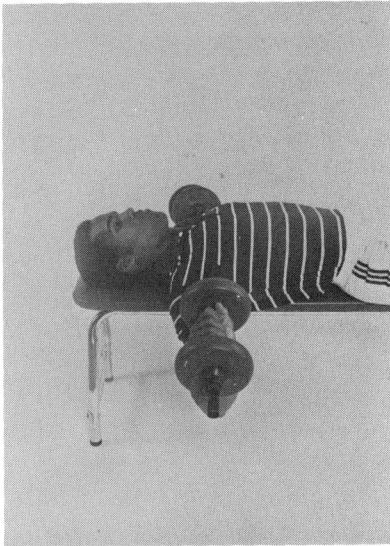

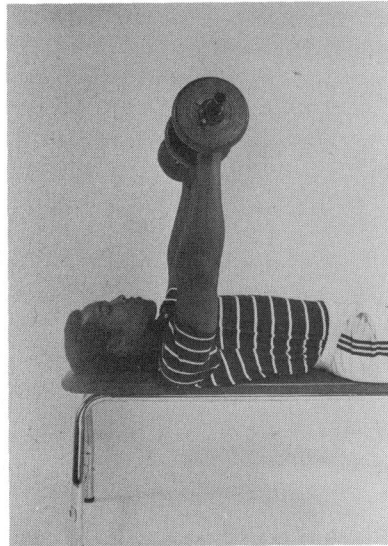

A variation of the dumbbell press is to use the bench. Dumbbells will allow you to discover strength differences between the arms.

the military press. Then press the dumbbells overhead until your arms are fully extended and the inner plates of the dumbbells are together. Bend your elbows and return the dumbbells to the starting position at shoulder height.

**What it does**: This is another deltoid exercise, with secondary emphasis on the triceps, pectorals and trapezius. The action of the dumbbell press is slightly different than either of the barbell press variations, however, because the arms are free to move using dumbbells and more muscle force is required to control the weights.

**Variations on a theme**: Variations are endless for dumbbell presses. For example, when you push the dumbbells up, rotate your hands as you go so that at the top of the movement your palms are facing one another. This twisting motion works the deltoids more directly. You can also start with your palms facing each other when the dumbbells are at shoulder height, twisting your hands so that your palms are facing forward at the top of the movement. Include some of these variations in form now and then in your workouts. Variety is the spice of life so an unexpected stimulation now and then will enhance your progress.

**Special considerations**: Dumbbell movements should be fluid and unhurried. Capitalize on the increased range of motion afforded by dumbbells. These presses can be done standing or seated. Remember that the dumbbell must be controlled at all stages of the movement.

## ARM EXERCISES
### Barbell Curls

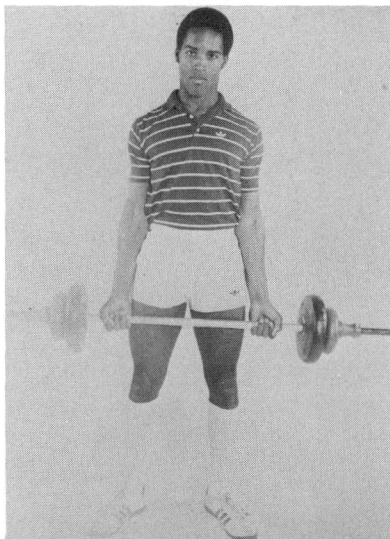

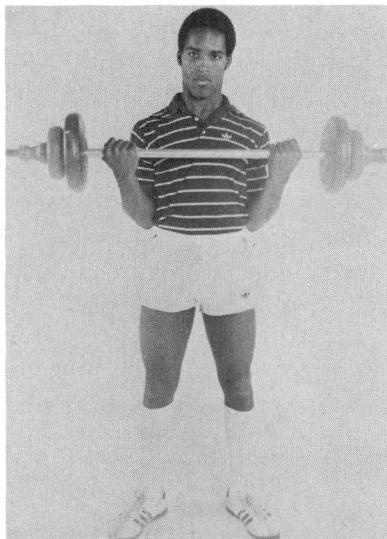

**Basic motion**: Stand erect with your feet shoulder-width apart and pointed slightly outward. Grasp a barbell with an underhand grip, your hands placed about shoulder-width apart, and your palms facing upward. Rest the barbell across the tops of your thighs as if you were near the finish of a deadlift. Hold your upper arms close to your sides and now raise the barbell in a semicircle from the tops of the thighs to your throat in a fluid motion, using only the strength of your biceps. Return along the same arc to the starting position, lowering the weight slowly and opposing gravity all the way.

**What it does**: The barbell curl is the number one exercise for the development of the biceps. The movement also works the brachialis muscle of the upper arm and the forearms.

**Variations on a theme**: Placing your hands nearer or farther apart than shoulder width affects your biceps differently. Placing your hands about a foot or less apart directs more force to the

**Barbell Curls**

Barbell curls are a basic exercise popular with bodybuilders. Avoid arching your back during the movement.

outsides of your biceps while taking a grip wider than shoulder width concentrates more force on your inner biceps.

**Special considerations**: Almost everyone is familiar with barbell curls, yet they are consistently done wrong. Most fail to concentrate the effort in the biceps. They are using their legs, shoulders, and just about every muscle but their biceps to help raise the weight. The movement should be slow and take about five seconds to complete one rep. Rushing the movement causes the barbell to swing like a pendulum, which gains momentum. To emphasize back rigidity, stand against a post or wall during the movement.

### Pulley Curls

**Basic movement**: Stand in front of the pulley station of the Universal Gym, facing the weight stack with your feet shoulder-width apart and about a foot back from the pulley. Point your toes slightly outward. Grasp the lower pulley handle with an underhand grip. Your hands should then be positioned about twelve to fifteen inches apart. Rest the pulley bar on your upper thighs in the same position a barbell would be at the start of the barbell curl. Pin your upper arms at your sides to restrict their movement and pull the pulley handle up in a semicircular motion from your thighs to your chin. Return to the starting position.

**What it does**: A pulley curl works the same muscles as a barbell curl—the biceps and the brachialis, with secondary emphasis on the forearm muscles.

**Variations on a theme**: Varying hand position on the pulley bar alters the exercise effect. Placing the hands less than one foot apart concentrates the effort in the outer portion of the biceps while a wide grip has more effect on the inner biceps.

**Special considerations**: Pulley curls on a Universal Gym are in some ways easier for the beginner than barbell curls, because there is less tendency to swing the body back and forth in an effort to develop momentum. Also, do not let the elbows drift outward, which takes the stress off the biceps and lets the shoulders do the work. Concentrate the effort in the biceps—feel the stretch and contraction and keep a steady, even pace.

### Reverse Curls

**Basic movement**: Take the same starting position as the barbell

## Reverse Curls

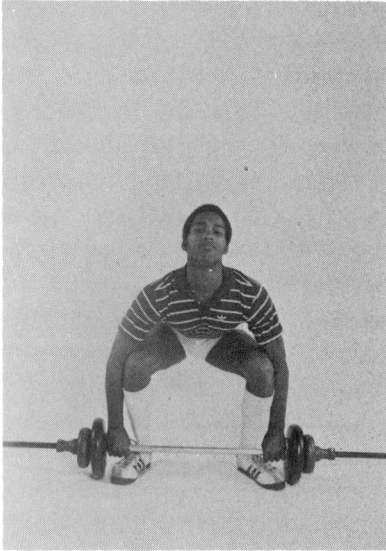

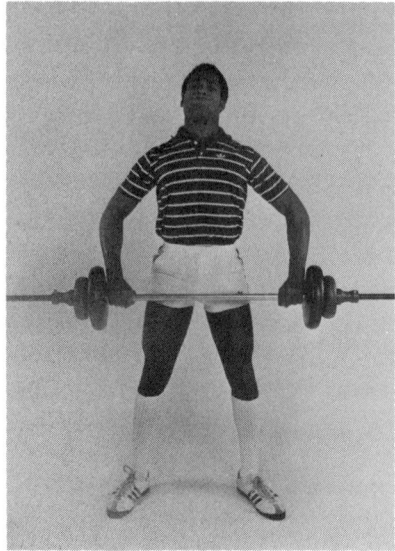

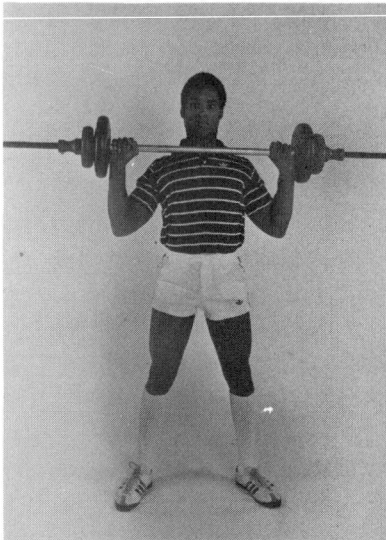

Reverse curls are difficult exercises. When lifting any weight, use the legs, keeping your back straight. This exercise works the brachialis muscle.

curl, except your palms should be faced toward, rather than away from your body. This overhand grip is called the reverse grip. With your arms pinned beside you, raise the barbell from your upper thighs to your chin in a semicircular motion and return along the same arc to the starting position.

**What it does:** Reverse curls are the most basic exercise for the brachialis muscle, which ties together the lifting motion of the biceps and the forearms. The wrist extensons play a secondary role in stabilizing the wrist position. The brachialis, which lies under the biceps, is an important muscle in many sports activities.

**Variations on a theme**: Many find that a grip in the center of the barbell with the index fingers about six inches apart is superior to a shoulder-width grip for isolating the exercise to the arms, rather than the shoulders. Try both grips to see which is more effective for you.

**Special considerations**: Keep the upper body straight and do not allow the elbows to drift away from the sides. This movement can also be done on the Universal Gym, although most find the use of free weights to be more effective.

### Seated Nautilus Curls

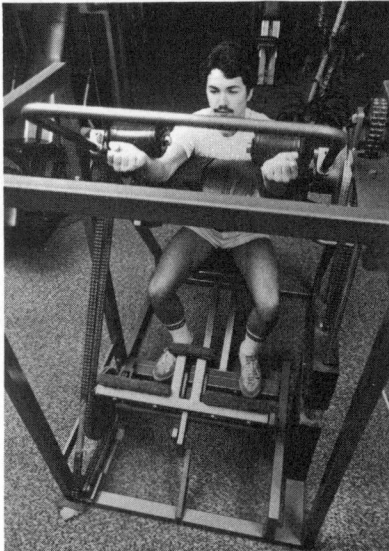

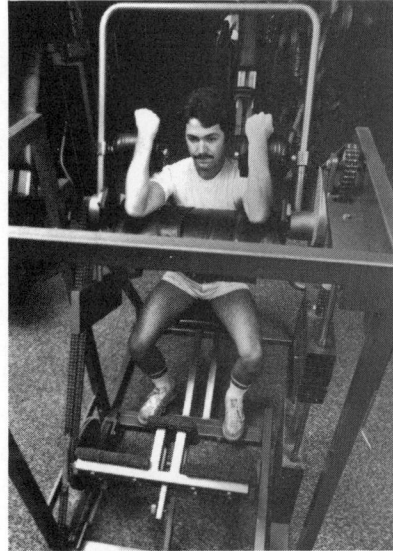

**Basic movement**: Position yourself in the Nautilus curl machine and adjust the seat height so that you can comfortably drape your arms over the angled padding, hands toward the bottom of the pads and the backs of your upper arms resting on the pads. After fastening the seat belt, push down on the foot pedals until you can slip your wrists under the small pads attached to the movement

**Seated Nautilus Curls**

Nautilus curls work the same muscles as the free weight exercise. Use the foot pedals to release your wrists when done.

arm. At the start of the movement, your wrists will be resting under the pads, your palms up, and your arms perfectly straight. Let go of the foot pedal to return resistance to your wrists. Curl the wrists up in a semicircular motion until you cannot raise them farther. Return to the starting position. Use the foot pedals to release your wrists when done.

**What it does**: Nautilus curls give the same training benefits as barbell curls or pulley curls for the development of the biceps and brachialis muscles.

**Variations on a theme**: Try curling the weight more slowly than usual and pausing for a count of three at the top of the movement. Then return to the starting position. You cannot use as much resistance with this variation, but it recruits the maximum possible number of muscle fibers.

**Special considerations**: As in all Nautilus exercises, the cam design will force the muscle to work during its entire motion. Do not defeat this beneficial effect by hurrying the motion.

### Lying Barbell Triceps Extensions

**Basic movement**: Lie on a bench with your head at one end and your feet on the floor at the other end of the bench. Get a narrow overhand grip (about six inches between hands) on a barbell that is resting on a rack at the end of the bench. Be sure to grip the bar at the balance points. Start with the barbell extended directly over your chest, your palms facing toward your feet and your arms perpendicular to the floor. Lower the barbell to your forehead in a semicircle by bending only your elbows and using the muscles of the back of your arms to control the weight. Return to the starting position with your arms fully extended above the chest and your elbows locked.

**What it does**: Triceps extensions are the best exercises for the development of the triceps muscles at the backs of the arms. The triceps work antagonistically to the action of the biceps in that they extend the arms, rather than flex them.

**Variations on a theme**: There are many ways to do triceps extensions with barbells and one of the best is called the French curl. Standing erect, with the barbell raised directly above the head and the arms fully extended, lower the bar as far behind the head as possible, keeping the upper arms motionless. This can best be done by forcing the elbows to the sides of the head as the

## Lying Barbell Triceps Extensions

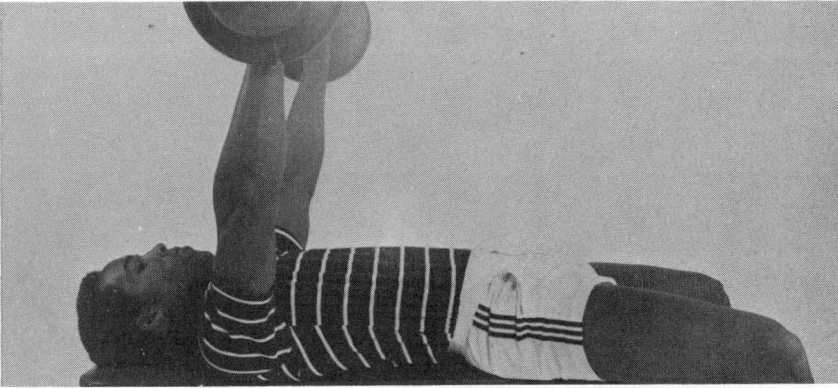

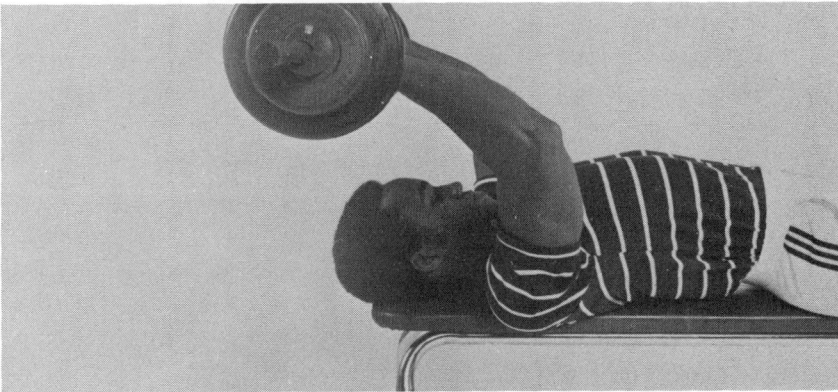

For the lying barbell triceps extension use a narrow grip. The palms of your hands should be facing toward your feet. Lower the barbell to your forehead.

weight is lowered and by gripping the barbell with a narrow, overhand grip.

**Special considerations**: Concentrate when doing this movement to direct the effort specifically at the triceps. Do not allow your shoulders to help in the movement and make sure that a fluid, fairly slow pace in each rep and set is maintained. This exercise depends on stretching as much as contraction for its beneficial effects. As in curling exercises, make sure that the elbows are not allowed to flare out at the sides during the movement, or unwittingly some of the stress will be taken off of the triceps.

## Dumbbell Triceps Extensions

**Basic movement**: Stand erect with your feet about shoulder-width apart and grasp a single dumbbell in both hands so that

## Dumbbell Triceps Extensions

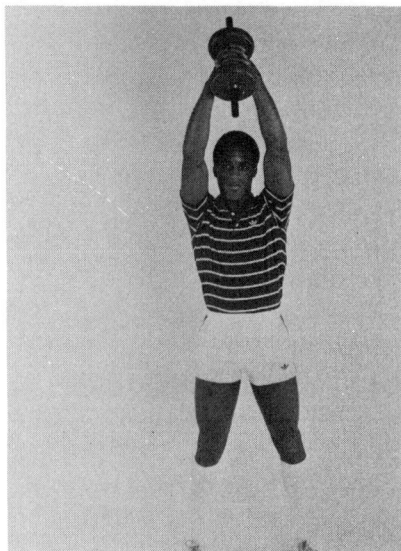

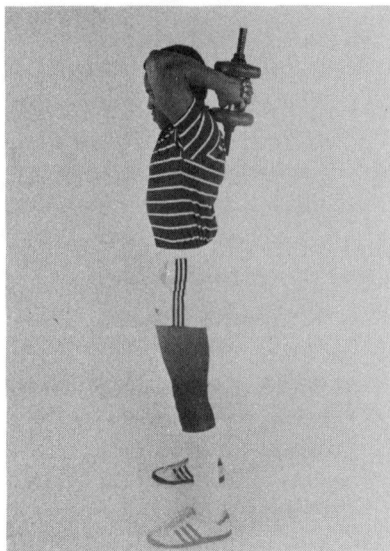

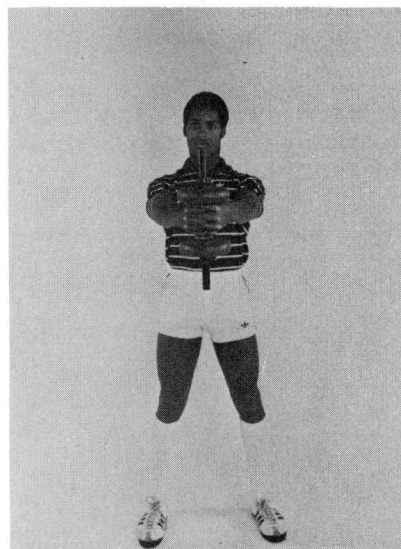

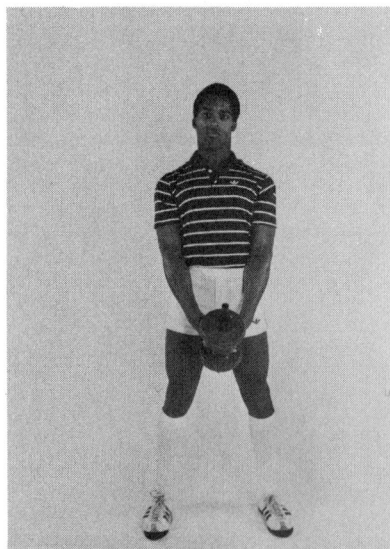

A dumbbell triceps extension begins with a dumbbell directly over your head, arms extended. This exercise works the triceps and the forearms. You can do the extensions using only one arm at a time.

your fingers are interlaced. Extend your hands directly over your head until your elbows are locked. The dumbbell handle should be perpendicular with the floor and both of your hands touching the underside of the top plate, while the bottom plate hangs down below your hands in a manner similar to the grip explained in the dumbbell pullover. Keep your upper arms stationary and bend your elbows to bend your arms in a semicircle until the dumbbell touches the back of your neck. Extend your arms back to the starting position using only the muscles of your triceps.

**What it does**: This variation of the barbell extension works the triceps and the forearms. Since the weight is better controlled than in the barbell extension, the tension on the shoulders is greater and provides an additional training effect.

**Variations on a theme**: Dumbbell triceps extensions can also be done with one arm at a time. Similarly, the exercise can be varied somewhat by holding one dumbbell in each hand. In either case, the movement is the same as that described earlier.

**Special considerations**: Make sure the elbows are not allowed to move away from the sides of the head. Get a complete stretch and full extension on every rep.

**Lat Machine Pushdowns**

**Basic movement**: Stand with your feet about shoulder-width apart and a foot or so from where the free weight or Universal Gym lat machine bar hangs down. Place your hands about six inches apart on the bar, assuming an overhand grip, palms facing the floor. Your hands should be placed right in the middle of the lat bar. Pull the bar down to the middle of your thighs so that your elbows are locked. Pin your elbows to your side and slowly bend your arms to full flexion, so that the bar travels in a semicircle from your thighs to your chin. Extend your arms, keeping your upper arms as stationary as possible, until the bar is again resting against your thighs. Repeat the movement as required.

**What it does**: Pushdowns work the triceps muscles, with secondary emphasis on the forearms.

**Variations on a theme**: By leaning inward toward the lat machine or Universal Gym, you put more tension on your triceps muscles. You will find this movement easier on your wrists if you keep them cocked, i.e., bent forward, throughout the movement.

**Special considerations**: This movement must be forced only by the triceps muscles. It is very easy to allow the shoulders or back to help out unless guarded against. Do the movement slowly and concentrate on keeping the upper arms motionless throughout.

### Nautilus Triceps Extensions

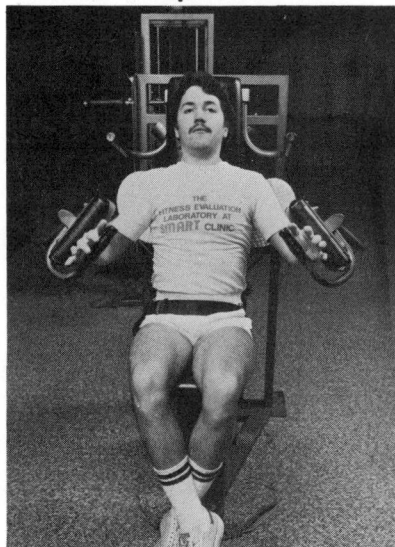

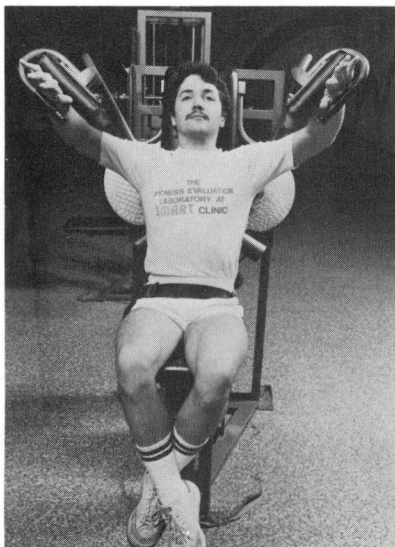

**Basic movement:** Adjust the seat of the Nautilus machine so that the backs of your upper arms are resting comfortably on the large lower pad. Place your hands against the smaller pads. Press the foot pedal down after you have buckled the seat belt. The extension apparatus will raise up so that you can rest your wrists against the small pads on the extension arm, palms open and facing each other. Let off the foot pedal to place the resistance on your wrists and bend your arms as far as they will go. When your arms are bent up as far as they will go, straighten them again using only triceps power. Return to the starting position and repeat as required.

**What it does:** The Nautilus machine is designed to concentrate the effort almost entirely on the triceps, with minimal help from the forearms.

**Variations on a theme:** You can also do this exercise with your palms facing away from one another to work your triceps from a slightly different angle.

**Special considerations:** Let the weights return fully over your head before you get off the machine. Pushing on the foot pedal will remove the resistance long enough for you to get your arms free.

## Nautilus Triceps Extensions

Nautilus triceps extensions isolate, almost totally, the effort in the triceps. You can also do this exercise with your palms facing away from one another.

## ABDOMINAL EXERCISES
### Leg Raises

**Basic movement:** Lie on your back on a slant board or at the sit-up board of the Universal Gym, and grasp the foot straps or rollers with your hands. Bend your legs at your knees to about a 30-degree angle. Raise your legs up until your knees come within about six inches of your face. Your legs should remain bent throughout. Lower your legs to the starting position and repeat as required.

**What it does:** This movement is excellent for the lower frontal abdominal muscles and the hip flexors of the thigh.

**Variations on a theme:** By changing the degree of slant on the sit-up or slant board, you can increase the difficulty of this movement. A more pronounced slant, up to about 45 degrees from the floor, increases the resistance noticeably.

**Special considerations:** Like all abdominal exercises, the movement should be slow and fluid. Take care not to arch the back. The bent-knee position in this and other abdominal movements is designed to reduce lower back strain.

### Sit-Ups/Crunches

**Basic movement:** You are already familiar with this movement from the freehand program. Lie on the slant board or the sit-up station of the Universal Gym. Place your feet under the foot straps or rollers and bend your knees at about a 30-degree angle. Interlace your fingers behind your head and curl your torso upward until your elbows touch your knees. Return in the same fashion to the starting position and repeat. The crunch is a similar exercise. Lie on your back perpendicular and next to a flat bench, resting your legs from your knees down on the bench, so that your upper thigh is pointing straight up to the ceiling. Interlace your hands behind your head and curl your torso upward as far as it will go. You will be unable to raise your torso completely up from this position, but you will feel the effort in your abdominals. Resting your legs on the bench reduces the potential use of your hip flexors in the movement.

**What it does:** The frontal abdominals, especially the upper abdominals, are worked, with some emphasis on the hip flexors.

**Variations on a theme:** As you curl your body upward, twist your body at your waist from left to right. This variation puts further tension on your abdominals. You can also vary the placement of your hands. Instead of locking them behind your head, you can cross them in front of your chest or place each hand around the side of your waist at the level of your hip bone.

**Special considerations**: When you perform the sit-up or crunch properly, your motion will be fluid and smooth. To curl your body upward, sequentially lift your torso up, starting with your upper back, then the middle of your back, and finally your lower back. Many novices jerk their bodies upward, thinking that this motion is somehow more efficient. But jerky motions are counter-productive because they take tension off your abdominals.

### Nautilus Knee Pullups/Knee-Ups

**Basic movement**: Although these exercises are done on different apparatus, their effects are identical, making them interchangeable.

**Nautilus**: Sit on the edge of the bench facing the moveable roller pad. After you fasten the seat belt around your waist, pull the roller up with your arms and slide your knees under the pads. Lie back, allowing the roller to descend with your legs and grasp the handles alongside your body to steady yourself. Raise your knees as far as you can and as close to your chest as they will go. Slowly lower your legs to the starting position and repeat.

**Free apparatus**: Sit on the end of a flat bench with your legs extending away from the end of the bench. Grasp the sides of the bench and lean your upper torso back at about a 45-degree angle. In this position your arms will be straight or slightly bent. Raise your feet off the ground a few inches, keeping your knees together and your legs straight. It helps to point your toes slightly. Slowly bend your knees toward your chest, keeping your upper torso motionless. When your knees touch your chest, they should be fully bent. Lower your legs in the same arc until they are fully extended again.

**What it does**: The knee-up in its various forms is an excellent conditioner of all of the frontal abdominal muscles and the hip flexors. Because the abdominals and hip flexors are so important in sports, you should train them from a number of different angles.

**Variations on a theme**: Some gyms have an apparatus for doing

## Nautilus Knee-Ups

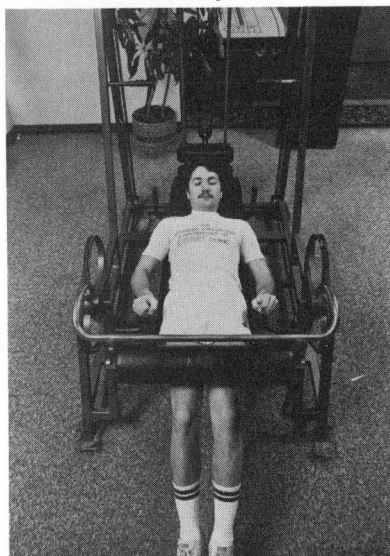

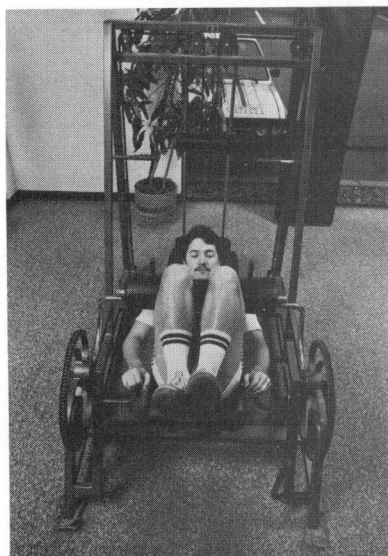

Lie on your back to start Nautilus knee-ups. Raise your knees as far as you can and as close to your chest as they will go.

knee-ups from a vertical position. You can also do them lying down on the same slant board you use to do sit-ups.

**Special considerations**: These exercises cause lower back pain in some individuals. If pain is felt in the lower back or a clicking sensation occurs there while doing either of these movements, discontinue knee-ups or knee pullups and return to standard sit-ups or knee pullups is that they do not require as much abdomin-ups or knee pull-ups is that they do not require as much abdominal strength as other abdominal exercises. They can be used to build strength for more difficult movements and are particularly useful for toning the lower abdomen, an area many women find especially hard to keep trim.

## LEG EXERCISES
### Squats/Lunges

**Basic movement**: You are already familiar with these exercises from the freehand program. Now you will be doing them with resistance provided by a barbell.

**Squats**: Standing with your feet about shoulder-width apart and your toes pointed slightly outward, place a barbell across your shoulders. Position the barbell behind your neck in such a way

## Squats

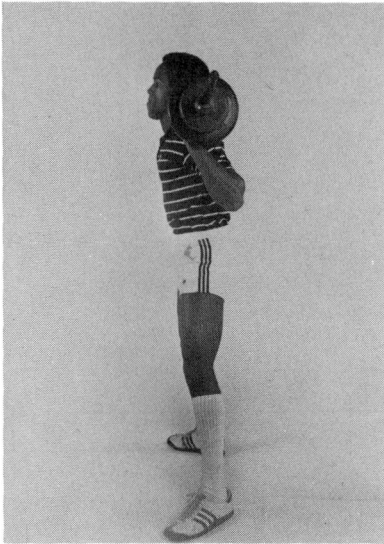
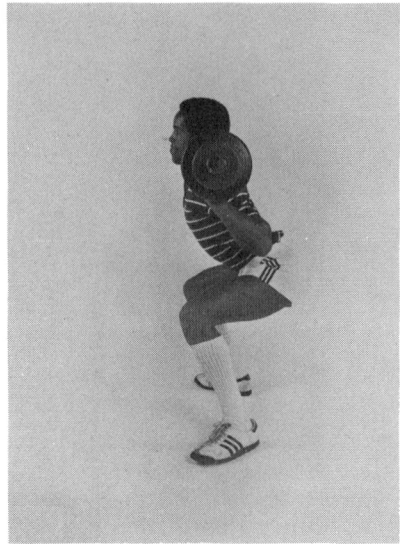

## Lunges

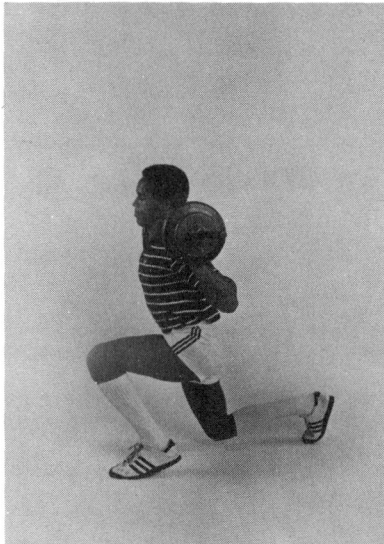

Never bounce at the bottom of a leg squat, because it strains the knees. Do not bend forward at the waist. Lunges call for you to throw one leg forward, your trailing leg bending slightly.

that you can balance it, grasping the bar with your palms facing outward and your hands near the plates. Keeping your upper body straight, bend at your knees and sink into a deep knee-bend until your thighs are parallel with the floor. Return to the upright position using only the power of your legs and buttocks.

**Lunges:** Assume the same starting position with the barbell as in the squat. Lunge forward with one leg, keeping your upper body straight. Your trailing leg will bend slightly at your knee and the heel of your trailing leg will then come up off the floor. Stretch in this position until the knee of your trailing leg touches the floor. Push yourself back up to the starting position using only the power of your forward leg and repeat the movement with your other leg lunging forward.

**What it does**: These basic movements are essential at all stages of development for training the thigh and buttocks muscles. The squat and lunge are essentially interchangeable, although many pursuits shun the lunge in favor of the squat. Other top body-builders feel that the lunge is a superior thigh conditioner, especially for women and those interested in defining and separating the thigh musculature. A good strategy for the beginner is to use the squat and lunge interchangeably on alternate days in the gym. Do not be concerned that the squat will develop the thigh muscles excessively. Most people with large thighs, especially women, notice a decrease in the size of their thighs after doing squats or lunges for a few months, because the muscle toning effect eliminates excess inches.

**Variations on a theme**: Many gyms have leg press machines that accomplish essentially the same thing as the squat. In this variation, you lie on your back and push against a stack of weights suspended above you by using your leg and buttocks muscles. Use the free weights for a while to get used to the exercise before moving to a machine. You want to get used to controlling the weights without assistance. Leg presses can also be done at the leg press station of the Universal Gym.

**Special considerations**: Never bounce at the bottom of either the squat or lunge, because this puts excessive strain on the ligaments of the knee and on the lower back. You should also develop a habit of wearing a weightlifting belt in both of these movements. Remind yourself not to bend forward at your waist in any part of the movement, which is a cause of lower back strain. Focus your eyes on a point somewhere in front of you as you do these movements and you will find it easier to keep your upper body straight.

Lighter weights will enable you to place the bar on your shoulders using only the strength of your arms. With heavier weights you will need to use the squat rack to hold the barbell in place as you position yourself under it. Do not attempt to use heavy weights in the squat without using the squat rack and without the assistance of a spotter or training partner. They are there to help in the event you have trouble handling the weight.

### Leg Extensions

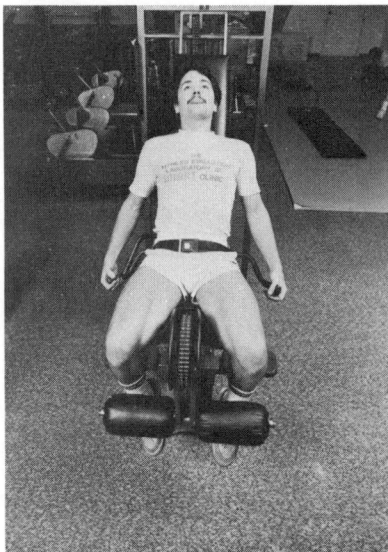

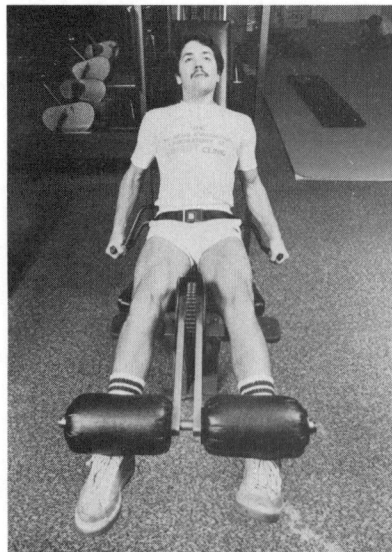

**Basic movement**: Leg extensions can be done using free weights, the Universal Gym, or a Nautilus machine.

**Free weights**: Sit on the edge of the free weight leg extension machine, hook the tops of your feet under the lower set of rollers, and steady your upper body by grasping the sides of the bench beside your hips.

**Universal Gym**: The starting position is the same as for the free-weight position.

**Nautilus**: Sit in the Nautilus machine and adjust the seat back by lifting the handle on the right side of the machine (some machines will not be adjustable) until your knees extend no more than one inch past the front edge of the bench. Place the tops of your feet under the single set of rollers on the machine. Fasten the lap belt, and grasp the handles at the sides of your hips to steady yourself.

The movement consists of extending your legs, using only the

### Leg Extensions

Leg extensions on the Nautilus begin with knees bent. Extend your legs slowly and completely, never using your momentum.

strength of your thighs, until your knees are locked. Pause at full extension for a second or so and then gradually lower your legs to their starting position.

**What it does**: Leg extensions that are done properly mainly involve the quadriceps, with minimal assistance from the arms, abdominals, and the upper and lower back. Those who experience lower back pain doing squats can substitute with leg extensions and the leg curl.

**Variations on a theme**: Alternate foot positions occasionally, doing some sets with the toes pointed inward or outward instead of with the feet parallel. Alternate sets can also be done using only one leg at a time.

**Special considerations**: This movement should be done slowly and completely, never allowing momentum to assist in either lifting or lowering the weight. Within a few weeks increased muscle definition in the thighs will be visible.

## Leg Curls

**Basic movement**: Leg curls compliment leg extensions. They can be done using free weights, the Universal Gym, or a Nautilus leg curl machine.

**Free weight or Universal**: Lie face down on the free weight leg curl table or the leg curl station of the Universal Gym, with your knees extending an inch or two past the edge of the bench. Hook your heels under the upper rollers and grasp the edge of the bench for stability. Allow your legs to straighten completely.

**Nautilus**: There will be only one set of rollers on the Nautilus leg curl machine, so lie down as on the free-weight machine and hook your heels under the rollers, grasp the handles at the sides of the machine, and lower your legs until they are fully extended.

Bend your legs as far upward toward your buttocks as you can by flexing them at the knee and using the power of your hamstring muscles. Lower to the starting position and repeat.

**What it does**: This movement primarily works the hamstrings, with secondary emphasis on the buttocks and calves.

**Variations on a theme**: Again, you can switch the positions of your feet as you did in the leg extension to work different parts of the hamstring muscle.

**Special considerations**: Remember when doing leg curls to keep your hips down when curling the rollers upward. If your hips are allowed to lift up, you rob the exercise of some of its range of motion.

## Leg Curls

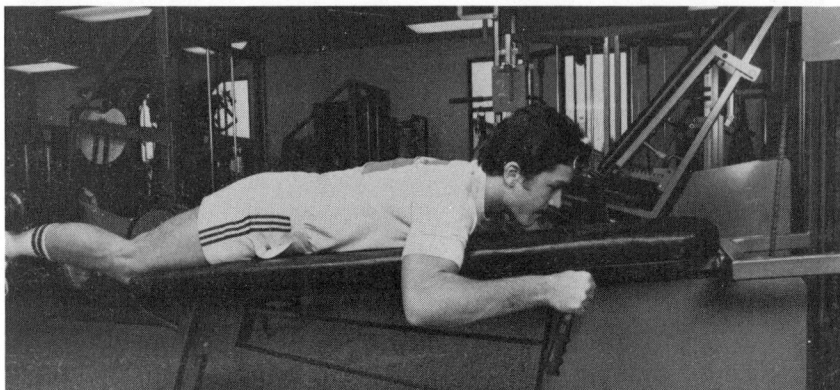

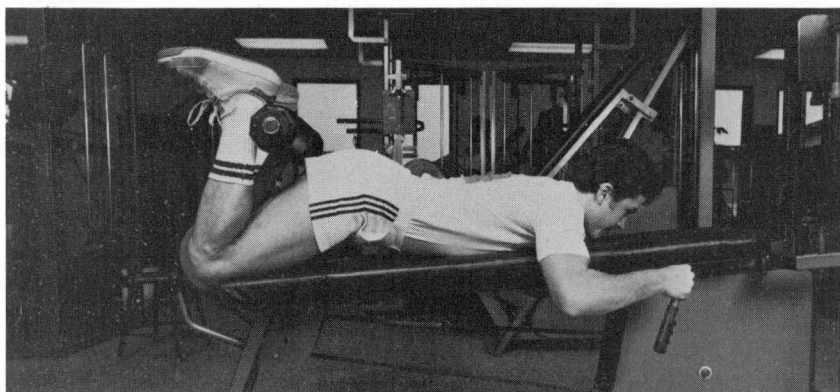

On the Nautilus leg curl machine begin with your legs extended, hands grasping the handles at your side. Bend your legs as far up toward your buttocks as you can by flexing them at the knee.

## Calf Raises

**Basic movement**: Stand with your feet shoulder-width apart and place a barbell on your shoulders in the same manner as you would for squats. Put the balls of your feet on a plank about four inches thick with your heels on the floor. Rise on your toes as far as you can and still retain your balance. Return to the starting position.

## Calf Raises

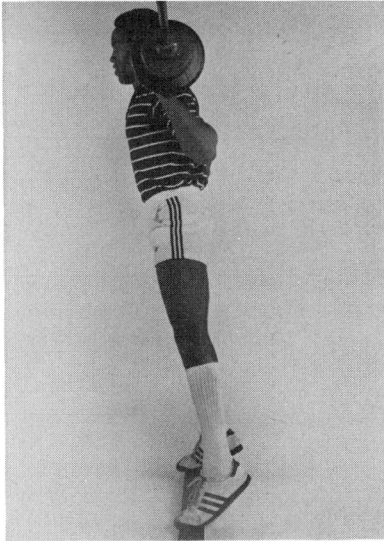

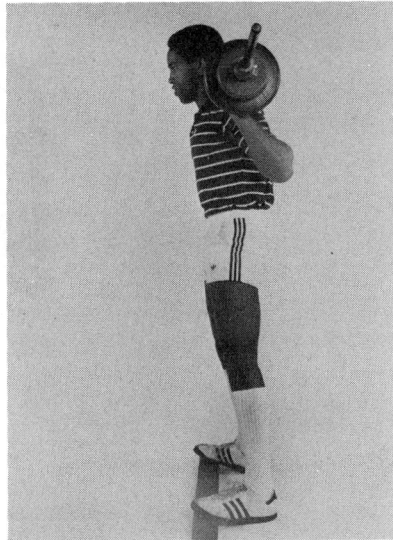

Calf raises are made more difficult with the addition of a barbell behind the neck. Strive to keep the calves straight at all times.

**What it does:** Calf raises work the calf muscles, especially the gastrocnemius and the soleus. The thighs, back, and abdominals offer some supporting resistance.

**Variations on a theme:** If your gym has a calf machine, you will find it easier to do calf raises on it, because the balance factor will be ameliorated. To do calf raises on the calf machine, stand in front of the machine and place your shoulders under the yolks. Stand on the block in front of the machine and raise up on your calves as far as possible, pushing up on the shoulder yolks. Another variation of calf raises, more properly called calf presses, can be done on the Universal Gym or on Nautilus calf machines. In either of these machines, sit in the seat at the leg press station, extend your legs with your feet on the pedals, and with your legs still extended, flex your toes up and down on the pedals. Use only your calf muscles. The beginner should do calf raises initially using free weights or a calf machine, because controlling the weight during the movement provides a valuable training effect, which is missing from the Universal Gym and Nautilus machine.

**Special considerations:** You must strive to keep your calves straight at all times, or they will end up working too much in the movement. Elevating the balls of your feet allows you to stretch your heels more completely than if your feet were flat on the floor. This stretch is particularly important for runners, who use their calf muscles extensively.

## SUPPLEMENTARY EXERCISES

We will include two exercises here that may be difficult to include in your program initially, but which are so valuable that you will want to include them, at least periodically, when you develop the stamina necessary to handle them in addition to the other basic movements.

### Parallel Bar Dips

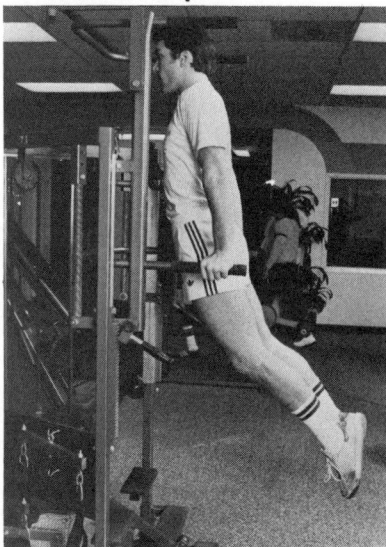

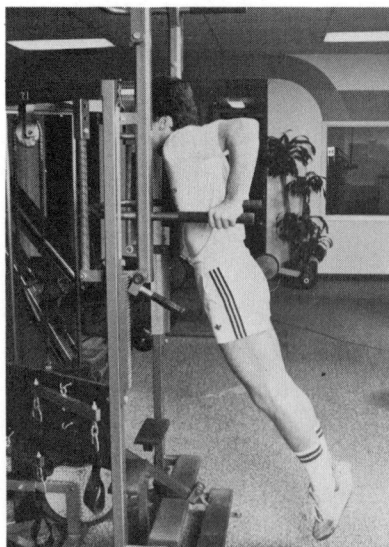

**Basic movement:** Grip the ends of a set of parallel bars or a set of bars on a specialized dipping apparatus so that your palms are facing one another. Jump off the floor and support your weight off the ground with your arms. If you have to, bend your knees so that your feet are completely off the floor. Keep your arms straight and along the sides of your body. Now bend your arms so that your elbows move back and your shoulders descend toward the bars. Lower your upper body in this manner as far as you can, pause there, and then press back up to the starting position. Pause

### Parallel Bar Dips

Begin parallel bar dips with your arms straight at your sides, grasping the handles. Lower your upper body as far as you can, pause, then press back up to the starting position.

at the top and repeat the movement.

**What it does**: Dips work the lower pectorals, the deltoids, and the triceps, with secondary emphasis on the upper pectorals and latissimus dorsi.

**Variations on a theme**: Leaning forward during the movement puts more resistance on the pectorals, while keeping the upper body erect forces the deltoids and triceps to carry more of the load. This exercise involves several muscle groups simultaneously, thus promoting fitness in muscles that function together in many athletic events.

**Special considerations**: Keep your elbows centered above the bars at all times. The movement should be fluid and relatively slow, so that you do not use momentum to assist you in lowering or lifting your body. Remember, the act of resisting the downward pull of gravity as you lower your body produces training effects as valuable as the pressing movement back up.

### Chinning

**Basic movement**: Jump up and grasp a high horizontal bar with your hands at shoulder width and your palms facing out. Allow yourself to hang down with your arms fully extended and your feet off the floor. Bend your legs at the knee if this will help to keep your feet off the floor. Pull yourself upward (feel the effort in the latissimus and shoulders) until your chin is just above the bar. Slowly lower yourself to the starting position and repeat.

**What it does**: Chinning is an integrative exercise that develops the latissimus dorsi, biceps, deltoids, and forearms.

**Variations on a theme**: There are numerous body positions that produce subtly different effects on the body. The width of your grip on the chinning bar varies the relative contribution of the latissimus. A wide grip will stretch the lats, while a narrow grip, about a foot between your hands, puts more of the effort on the upper back, shoulders and arms. If you grip the bar so that your palms are facing toward you, you will attack your biceps directly as well as exercise the biceps-deltoid functional tie-in. The body moves because of the interaction of different muscle groups, so these tie-in movements are excellent for overall conditioning. Similarly, using a wide grip with your palms facing outward, you can bring your body up until the back of your neck touches the bottom of the bar. This variation works the frontal deltoids, as evidenced by the pump you will get in your shoulders.

**Special considerations**: Be sure to arch your back and force your elbows back in this movement for maximum stretch.

## BASIC ROUTINES

The following programs are suggested routines using the basic exercises. You need not feel confined to these specific exercises. Feel free to adapt a workout to suit your needs. You may not be able to complete three sets of each exercise in these programs right away, even if you spent some time in the freehand program before coming into the gym. In that case, try starting out doing one good set of each movement and gradually work up to three as your fitness level increases. However, you should strive for eight to ten good reps in each exercise before adding sets. Optional exercises in each program are those that you should try to work into your regimen when you feel strong enough to handle them.

Each of these progressive resistance programs should be preceded by ten minutes of warmup. After completing whatever program you choose, spend ten minutes in warmdown.

### FREE WEIGHT PROGRAM (3 SETS EACH)

Bench press
Bent rowing
Parallel bar dips (optional)
Dumbbell pullovers
Chins (optional)
Deadlifts (optional)
Military press
Barbell curls
Reverse curls
Barbell triceps extension
Sit-ups/crunches
Bent-leg raises
Squats/lunges
Calf raises

## UNIVERSAL GYM PROGRAM  (3 SETS EACH)

Bench press
Lat machine pulldowns
Seated press
Chins (optional)
Pulley curls
Lat machine pushdowns
Sit-ups
Bent-leg raises
Leg press
Leg curls
Calf presses

## NAUTILUS PROGRAM

(Note: Since these machines are designed to give you a really intense workout, never do more than two sets of any Nautilus exercise in *any* beginning program.)

Bench presses
Pullovers
Seated press
Curls
Triceps extensions
Knee pullups
Leg extensions
Leg curls
Calf press

## FREE WEIGHT/NAUTILUS COMBINED PROGRAM (FREE WEIGHTS–3 SETS)

Bench press (barbell)
Nautilus pullovers
Nautilus seated press
Barbell curls
Dumbbell triceps extensions
Sit-ups/crunches
Nautilus leg extensions/curls
Calf machine raises

## FREE WEIGHT/UNIVERSAL GYM COMBINED PROGRAM
## (3 SETS BOTH VARIATIONS)

Barbell bench press
Bent rowing
Lat pulldowns
Dumbbell pullovers (optional)
Parallel bar dips
Seated press (Universal)
Barbell curls
Reverse curls (optional)
Barbell triceps extensions
Bent leg raises
Squats/lunges (you may substitute Universal
leg presses/curls if so desired)
Calf machine raises

## FREE WEIGHT/UNIVERSAL GYM/NAUTILUS
## COMBINED PROGRAM

Perhaps the best situation you could encounter—doing three
sets each of free weight and Universal movements and no more
than two sets of Nautilus machine exercises.
Barbell bench press
Lat pulldowns
Nautilus pullovers
Dumbbell press (may use military press instead)
Parallel bar dips (optional)
Barbell curls
Barbell reverse curls
Lat machine pushdowns
Chins (optional)
Sit-ups/crunches
Bent-leg raises
Squats/lunges
Nautilus leg curls
Calf machine raises
These programs will work the various major muscle groups of
the body in a unified, integrated manner. Do not feel confined,
however, to specific parts of these programs. For example, you
may get a better effect from doing dumbbell pullovers than you

do from the same movement on the Nautilus pullover machine. Similarly, you may want to include deadlifts in your program instead of bent rowing. You can experiment a bit to see what works best for you.

As noted earlier, whatever beginning program you choose should be completed in an hour or less, including warmdown. Keeping a brisk pace will increase the cardiovascular benefits of the progressive-resistance exercises. You will find it difficult at first to combine heavy aerobic exercise with three workouts per week in the gym. Increase your workload slowly, but try to put in two sessions of running or swimming each week. At first you may want to include about 15 minutes of jogging or swimming as part of your warmdown. If you are already a runner, it is easy to overtrain by combining too much running with your heavy gym training. If you feel fatigued on your rest days, you are probably training a bit too hard. Listen to your body.

After the warmdown, use the sauna or whirlpool, if your gym has one. Keep in mind the cautions I mentioned previously about the use of these facilities. Never stay in the sauna more than fifteen minutes, particularly if you have lost a lot of fluids during the workout. And fluid lost during the workout should be made up as soon as possible, preferably a little at a time during the workout itself. After your sauna, shower down, taking care not to plunge into cold water immediately after stepping out of the sauna. After your shower, you should feel superb, ready to take on the world and hungry for your next workout. If you don't enjoy yourself, it really isn't worth doing; feel good about your progress!

## HINTS ON TRAINING IN THE GYM

Three workouts per week are optimal in the beginning gym program, just as in the freehand program. If you absolutely cannot work out three times per week, you can still make progress on two workouts each week. To accomplish all of the exercises, garner maximal cardiovascular training effects, and gain strength and flexibility from progressive resistance sets, you should move from set to set and exercise to exercise briskly, taking no more than one minute rest between sets. Longer rest periods are counterproductive because they allow the heart rate to slow and the muscles to stiffen. Keep your pulse rate above 130 beats per minute fairly constantly, even between sets if possible.

You must expect a fair share of muscular soreness after the workout, particularly the day after the workout early in your tenure in the gym. Don't be afraid of soreness—it means growth. Some soreness and stiffness means that you worked the muscles hard enough in the last workout to effect training benefits. Your body will recuperate and come back stronger. We emphasized in the freehand program the importance of recuperation to achieve progress. It becomes doubly important in the gym training programs because you are placing even greater demands on your body. The day of rest between gym workouts is absolutely essential, as is adequate sleep and proper nutrition. As you get used to the gym program, you will be able to run, swim, or engage in other sports activities on your so-called rest days, but do not go overboard. Overtraining is a malady that has only recently been given its proper due in the world of sportsmedicine. It can affect both the novice and Olympic champion. The early symptoms of overtraining include appetite loss, insomnia, a rapid pulse when you get up in the morning, and a general feeling of fatigue and lack of interest in training, schoolwork, or business. When you exert your body repeatedly beyond the point that it can recuperate, it begins to break down. The overtrained athlete is more prone to injury and infection. You will not make progress in any athletic program while in this state. The only known cure is to cut back for a while in training, get plenty of rest, and wait for your drive to improve and the old spark of life to return. To prevent overtraining, keep up with your training log and self-assessment techniques.

Although gym training is a safe sports activity when conducted properly, injuries are nonetheless a part of the athletic experience and they could happen to you. Bruises and abrasions occur occasionally in the gym but aside from basic first aid, these should cause no major problems. Muscle strains or pulls are another matter entirely. Do not confuse normal stiffness and soreness with more serious injuries. A muscle strain can be painful enough to prevent you from training, but generally, such strains can be worked out by doing a full and complete warmup before the workout. A muscle pull, on the other hand, involves the actual tearing of muscle tissues. Your only recourse is to see a doctor, who will prescribe complete rest and inactivity for the affected body part. After a period of rest you can gradually begin working the muscle again. Nonetheless, a pulled muscle can be serious and should be brought to the attention of a physician. The first aid for either a muscle strain or pull is similar. Ice should be packed on the body part immediately after injury to reduce swelling. Ice packs also keep the muscle from cramping and further damage by that means. Anything but the most minor strains should be diagnosed by a physician immediately.

Next to muscle strains, the most common weight training injuries involve back problems. The spine is often the weak link in the human body, because man's erect stance compresses his spinal column, resulting in degeneration of the disks between the vertebrae, as well as pinched nerves. Generous use of spinal stretching exercises, such as hanging from a chinning bar, will help, as will the use of a weightlifting belt.

The best course against all muscle and joint injuries is sufficient warmup prior to lifting a heavy weight. If you warm up properly, your chances are better that you will never experience anything more severe than a simple muscle strain in the gym. Should you have a persistent back pain see a physician promptly.

## PROGRESSION—HOW LONG TO STAY ON THE BASIC PROGRAM AND WHERE TO GO FROM THERE

As you work up to three sets of free weight and Universal machine exercises and two sets of Nautilus exercises, you will probably find that after a time the weight you are using for 8 to 10 reps seems to be too easy. Once you can do those three sets, the last two reps of every movement should be really tough, because that's where the potential for growth occurs. You may then add a little weight to each movement, perhaps only five pounds or so, so that 8 reps is again challenging. Work up to 10 reps, then add a little more weight, and so on. That is where the "progressive" in progressive resistance training comes from—progressively giving your body a little more stimulation, staying hungry for more, and adapting to a higher fitness level a little at a time. Your muscles must be slightly overloaded, then given time to adapt.

During the basic program you will see incredible changes in your body. You will notice muscles you never thought you had. Your fitness level in all four of the components of fitness will be markedly elevated. You will become leaner and will look and feel terrific. The basic program, including warmup and warmdown will consume between 500 and 800 calories, depending on your body mass, sex, and intensity. Thus, since one pound of body fat contains about 3500 calories, you will lose perhaps a pound of fat every two weeks or so just from the basic program, assuming your caloric intake does not increase. Add aerobic activities on one or two non-gym training days per week, and you see even greater changes in your body fat percentage. Even if you are overweight, you should not try to lose more than a pound or two a week, especially while training, because you will be weakened and unable to put full effort into each gym session. In addition, more rapid weight loss means that you are cutting calories severely. You may not be getting essential nutrients from the reducing regimen.

While you will lose body fat as a consequence of the gym training program, assuming you do not increase your food intake, that fat loss may or may not be reflected in a change in body weight. Remember that muscle tissue is denser, more compact than fat. Women, especially, may find that their weight stays relatively static, although their measurements will improve dramatically. It is not uncommon for you to actually gain weight on the gym program while simultaneously losing significant amounts of body fat. The added weight is functional muscle tissue. Do not be concerned with weight per se; the amount of fat matters, so let your body fat levels be your guide.

Once beyond the level of the beginning gym trainee, you will begin the types of specialized gym exercises designed to work individual muscle groups, to refine the body. The emphasis will be on increased intensity, so your body must be ready for the greater workload.

How can you tell when you have gone beyond the beginning and into the intermediate training level? There are several guidelines. First, at the end of the beginning program you will have about doubled your strength and endurance, handling nearly twice the weight in each exercise as you were capable of at the start. You can do five or six sets per body part. Second, the male will find that the circumference of his chest has become 8 to 10 inches greater than that of his waist. Third, both the male and female will note profound changes in the visibility of muscle groups under the skin, partly due to the increased size of each muscle group.

The time you will need to spend on the basic gym program varies, according to your initial condition and your own physiology. A highly fit individual may find that he is ready to move on to more difficult programs after only three months or so, while some people may require a year or more of training to develop the foundation for further progress. Remember, this is no contest; you are only interested in training for yourself. You may decide, in fact, that the changes you see in your body after several months on the basic program are in accord with your initial goals, and that you wish no further development. If this is the case, you can maintain this high level of fitness indefinitely simply by staying on the basic program.

If you want to continue your progress into intermediate and advanced training, the succeeding chapters will show you how.

# 6

# Intermediate Gym Techniques and Programs

The main differences between beginning-level and intermediate/advanced gym training are in the intensity of exercises and in the concentration on various individual muscles, rather than large muscle groups. Some new exercises will be introduced in this chapter to add to your routines, but the emphasis is on technique. By the time you reach the intermediate training level, you will have become an expert on knowing your body. You will know how to use a new exercise and incorporate it into your program. There are literally hundreds of intermediate- and advanced-level gym exercises and it is beyond the scope of this book to provide you with an overview of all of these. The intermediate or advanced trainee will want to keep abreast of these various exercises and of new techniques by reading further in the field.

## INTERMEDIATE TRAINING TECHNIQUES

### Gaining Additional Fitness/Strength Without Increasing Body Weight

Athletes in many sports that stress weight economy and those simply interested in progressing in the gym without adding muscle size and bulk can accomplish their goals easily. The key to gaining strength and muscular fitness without increasing body weight is to lower the number of reps in each set to three or less per set, while using weights in the range of 80 to 90 percent of your maximum ability for a single rep in each exercise. By now you will have a good idea what your maximum lift is in each movement. Then calculate which weights constitute 40, 60, 75, and 90 percent of this maximum figure. You will want to be especially careful in your warm-up activities, since the risk of muscle injury in near-maximal lifts is proportionately greater.

Following the warmup, you will want to do your sets in each exercise in approximately the following format:

    1 x 3 (one set of three reps) at 40 percent of your maximum
    1 x 3 at 60 percent
    1 x 2 at 75 percent
    3 x 1 at 90 percent (three sets of one rep each)

In the next workout, try to do four sets of one rep each at the 90 percent level, then five sets the following workout. Once you can do five sets at 90 percent of maximum, with one rep in each set, add 5 to 10 pounds of weight in all of the sets and drop back down to three sets at the 90 percent level. By working sets and weights in this manner, your strength and muscular fitness will increase rapidly with minimal weight increases. This is a tiring routine, so avoid overtraining.

### Split Routines

As long as you include a day of rest between workouts, you can begin to work out four days a week, if you desire. To do this efficiently, you will need to split your body in half, concentrating on one half of the body in one workout and the other half in the next, so that your entire body is worked twice in any given week. There are several ways to accomplish this so-called "split routine." The most common variation is to work your upper body and your lower body on alternate days. Another variation is to work your torso (chest, shoulders, upper back, abdominals) on one day and your arms and legs on alternate days. The split routine is advantageous because you will find it difficult to maintain sufficient energy in intermediate or advanced programs to work the whole body in any single workout. Split routines are also valuable for athletes currently engaged in other sports, because the threat of overtraining is lessened if the work is spread over longer periods of time. You can really set up the split routine in any way you like as long as you train functionally associated muscles together in the same workout. This means that you train either upper/lower body muscles on alternate days, pushing/pulling muscles on alternate days, and so on. The best way to plan the split routine is to work out on a Monday/Thursday, Tuesday/Friday schedule, thus allowing a full day of rest in the middle of the week and a free weekend to do whatever you like without worrying about being in the gym. Unlike the beginning programs, it is not necessary to have a full day of rest before doing any gymwork, just a day of rest between workouts using the same muscles.

### Varying Sets and Reps for Variety

In intermediate programs, you will find it necessary to change your routine slightly from time to time, so that, even if you are doing the same exercises, you are doing them in slightly different ways. Progress beyond the beginning levels will be harder to come by because the body will demand proportionately more stimulation in order to be forced to grow and adapt. The easiest way to do this is to change the number of sets or reps that constitute each movement, so that the body is constantly presented with new and different stimuli.

There are several possible strategies in this approach. As a beginning trainee, you consistently performed 8 to 10 reps of each movement, with a fixed amount of resistance in each set. As an intermediate, you are ready to alter this cycle. You can drop the reps down to 4 to 6 per set, and progressively add a bit more weight on each set. Thus, you might start out with a set of bench presses using 60 pounds of weight on the bar, which might represent 50 percent of your maximum press. During the next set you would jump the weight up to 70 pounds, again doing 4 to 6 reps. The third set might consist of 4 to 6 reps with 80 pounds. This scheme will give you an outstanding pump and will produce strength gains proportionately faster than doing identical sets.

Alternately, you can reduce the weight in succeeding sets, increasing the reps as you go along, so that in the last set, you are using perhaps 50 percent of your maximum poundage and doing perhaps 15 reps. Either of these variations is effective. Each one will produce that training effect most desired in any intermediate/advanced routine—the complete exhaustion of a given muscle group. To progress in the gym beyond the beginning level of competence, it will become increasingly important to work each muscle group to the point of failure. That is, the last set of any given movement must be virtually impossible to complete without assistance from a spotter, if you are using free weights. Hence, the value of a training partner becomes even more evident than it was earlier. Unless the muscle group being worked is trained to exhaustion, the recruitment of muscle fibers will be incomplete and the training stimulus will by definition be insufficient to force the body to adapt to a higher fitness level.

There is one important corollary to the principle of set and rep variation that can be useful for all intermediate/advanced trainees, regardless of their individual goals. In this variation, the last set of a given movement is called the *pump set*. In a pump set, you drop the weight down significantly, attempting to do a very high number of repetitions, generally 15 to 20. The pump set usually follows two sets with normal (6 to 10) reps using moderate weights. It will totally exhaust the muscle group being trained with little danger of injury, and is particularly effective on the large muscle groups, like the legs and chest, which require a great deal of work to become exhausted.

The number of reps done in a given set will affect the type of development the exercise will produce. If you desire improvement in strength and fitness without large increases in muscle bulk, keep your rep range on the high side, i.e., 12 to 15 reps per set, or follow the special technique on gaining strength without bulk given at the beginning of this chapter. If, on the other hand, you want to increase your lean body weight dramatically for sports such as football, where body weight is an asset, you should generally work in the range of 4 to 6 reps per set in each movement. Again, these considerations are not constants. Each person will respond differently to exercise and variations therein. You must be the final judge, trying a variation for a month or two and evaluating what it does or does not do for you. If you decide to move exclusively in the direction of low or high rep sets, remember that you must adjust the resistance in each exercise accordingly, so that the last few reps are very difficult.

It would be nice if you could still have a set program that would guarantee success no matter what your individual goals, but as an intermediate or advanced trainee, these guidelines would only serve as suggestions. Your evaluation of your own progress must be the basis for your future development. The intermediate exercises presented in this section are virtually foolproof, but the program that you decide to follow from here must be highly individualistic. We stressed earlier the importance of body awareness and self-evaluation techniques. Now you will increasingly rely on your own judgment to tell you what you want or need to do next. Continue to monitor your progress using the mirror as a tool and you will proceed to make unbelievable changes in your physique and overall fitness. Whatever your individual goals, you must increasingly rely on variety to continue to make progress. Many advanced strength training athletes change their programs at least slightly, even markedly, every few weeks or so; some never do exactly the same workout twice in a row. While you do not need so radical an approach to your program, variety is important to keeping the mind and body hungry for more.

## INTERMEDIATE EXERCISES AND SPECIFIC MUSCLES

In the intermediate exercise, you will be concentrating the effort of the movement on a specific muscle or muscle groups. The intermediate program will consist of the basic movements you learned in the beginning programs and some of these more specialized movements. We will increasingly isolate a muscle, working it from a number of different angles. This approach will be important for those of you interested in sports proficiency, because you will have more freedom to work on those muscles vital to your sport. Nonetheless, you will always continue to do the basic movements designed to attack the large, functional muscle groups.

As in any exercise program, the warmup is fundamentally important prior to beginning the progressive resistance portion of the program. The speed of the workout will also continue to develop cardiovascular endurance, but you will still want to include running or swimming on off-days. Many intermediate strength training athletes neglect the aerobic portion of the unified program and find that while their strength may increase, they tire more easily during hard workouts. Keeping up with aerobic training routines will prevent this from happening to you. The warmups, warmdowns, and aerobic training are also important from the standpoint of maintaining your flexibility and suppleness. You must always stretch the muscles after contracting them vigorously in the gym program, or you risk injury or muscleboundness.

Intermediate and advanced exercises rely more on free weights and less on the Universal Gym or Nautilus machines. Because of the limited range of variation in these machines, you can only improve so much by training on them exclusively. Most of the intermediate free-weight exercises are effective because they force your body to control the weight being used as well as lifting or lowering it.

## INTERMEDIATE GYM EXERCISES

### CHEST EXERCISES
### Incline/Decline Bench Press

**Basic movement:** In the incline press, lie on a 45-degree incline bench with your feet flat on the floor. Take a shoulder-width grip on the barbell. Hold the bar as you would for the normal bench press, with your palms facing away from your body and press the bar upward until your elbows are locked. Slowly lower the barbell to the level of your upper chest and repeat. The decline press is performed in the same manner, using a 30-degree decline bench. Lie back on the bench so that your head is at the lower end and your feet are hooked over the top of the bench. Assume the same grip on the barbell as in the incline press and alternately press and lower the weight. This same movement can be done at the bench press station of the Universal Gym, along with the incline press, if you so desire, but you will not get the benefit of controlling the weight that you do with free weights.

**What it does:** An incline press isolates the muscles of the upper pectorals, while the decline press similarly isolates the lower pectorals. Both movements work the triceps and the deltoids as well.

**Variations on a theme:** In either the incline or decline press, you can alter your grip spacing on the barbell to change the effect of the movement, just as you did in the standard bench press.

**Special considerations:** The movement should be smooth and relatively slow. You may want to use a spotter at first until you get used to controlling the weights. Incline presses are particularly valuable for athletes in sports like football where upper body pushing strength is especially important, because the exercise develops the chest and shoulder muscles, as well as the triceps, at the same angle that they are used in sports. Make sure you keep your elbows directly under the barbell when doing these movements, so that the stress is placed primarily on the pectoral muscles rather than the arms.

### Dumbbell/Nautilus Flies

**Basic movement**: Lie on a flat bench with your feet on the floor and grasp a dumbbell in each hand. Bend your elbows slightly and lower your arms to the sides so that your hands are almost down to the floor on either side of the bench. Now raise your arms in a circular motion, keeping your elbows slightly bent, until the dumbbells are positioned over your chest, with your arms fully extended. The movement should not be one of pressing the weights; rather, you should push the weights up and in front of you, as if you were hugging a big tree. You really want to feel the stretch in the pectoral muscles in this movement. Flies can also be done on the Nautilus chest machine. In this variation, you sit in the machine and place your forearms on the moveable pads out

### Dumbbell Flies

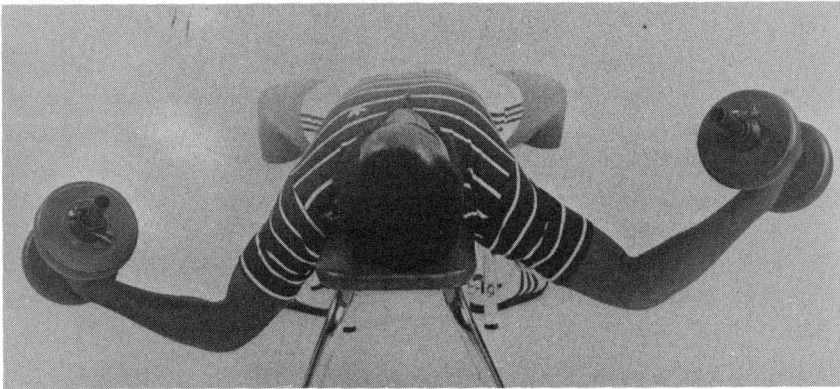

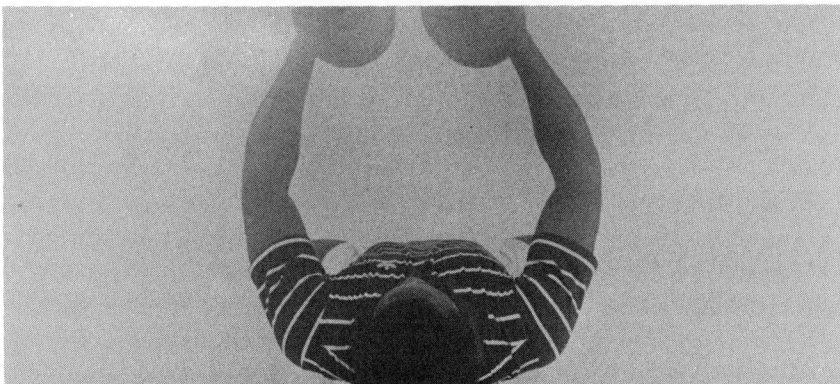

For the dumbbell flies, grasp the weights on the floor and lift them in a circular motion. You should push the weights up and in front of you, as if hugging a big tree.

## Nautilus Flies

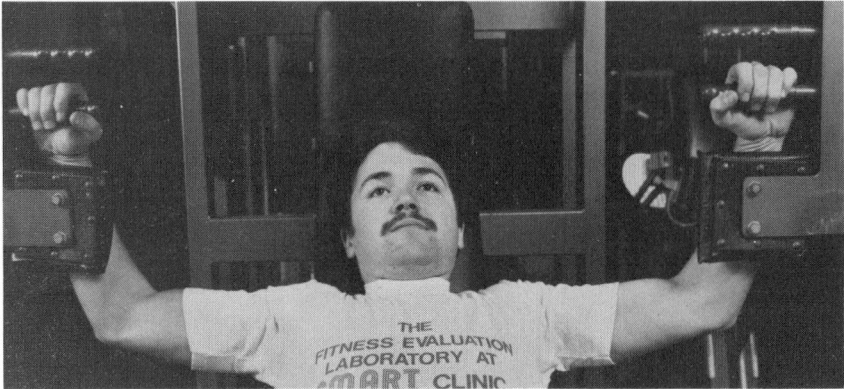

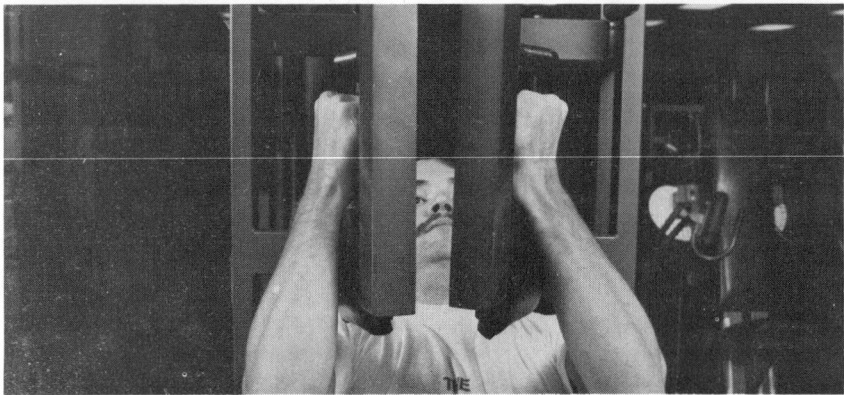

Nautilus flies begin with elbows extended, then bring them together. On the Nautilus machine hold the pads together for a few seconds at maximal contraction.

to your sides, grasping either the top or bottom set of horizontal handles attached to the pads. Your arms will then be parallel with the floor and stretched out as far behind your body as possible. Push the pads forward and inward with your elbows until they touch in the middle. Return to the starting position and repeat.

**What it does**: Flies are the number one isolation exercise for the pectoral muscles. Properly done, they will separate the fibers of the chest muscles, especially where they attach to the sternum. You virtually cannot achieve definition in the chest muscles without doing flies. Women find them especially useful because they develop the muscles that underlie the breasts, helping to retard sagging.

**Variations on a theme**: The fly can be done on either the flat bench or the incline or decline benches. The effect on the pectorals is then modified in a manner similar to that noted in the incline or decline presses.

**Special considerations**: Bending your elbows slightly will take the pressure off your elbow joints. The motion should always be a sweeping semicircle, akin to wrapping your arms around a large tree, rather than a pressing movement, which we have already done in other exercises. To increase the force on the pectorals, tense your muscles and really force the dumbbells upward when you have brought them in front of your chest and hold that position for a few seconds. Similarly, on the Nautilus machine, hold the pads together for a few seconds at maximal contraction.

### Parallel Bar Dips

We have already described this movement in the basic program, so we won't repeat it here. You should include them as an integral part of your intermediate program.

### BACK EXERCISES
### Power Cleans

**Basic movement**: Walk up to a barbell, place your feet about shoulder-width apart, bend down and grasp the barbell with an overhand grip. Keep your elbows straight, bend your knees, and lower your upper body toward the floor until your upper thighs are about parallel with the ground. Arch your back slightly by tensing your spine muscles and remain faced forward during the movement. In an explosive action, straighten your legs to begin the barbell movement off the floor. Keep your elbows locked and your arms straight so that they only act as cables to hook the barbell to your shoulders. As your legs straighten, begin extending your hips. When your entire body is erect, the barbell should be resting on the fronts of your thighs. Follow through on the pulling motion by rising on your toes and bending your elbows to swing the weight up to your shoulders, at which point you can move your elbows under it and let the bar settle across your deltoids at the base of your neck. Lower the weight by reversing the sequence by which you raised it and repeat as required.

**What it does**: Power cleans involve all of the back muscles, plus the thighs, buttocks, calves, biceps, and forearms. The name power clean tells you what this exercise does; it develops explosive power in all of the lifting muscles of your frame. Thus, while it is not an isolation exercise like most intermediate movements, it is an important part of the intermediate program, especially for those interested in the development of power.

**Variations on a theme**: The only real variation in this movement is to vary the weight used, from very heavy to light, so that you must really work to explode upward with the heavy barbell. Use the light weights to do one final pump set at the end.

**Special considerations**: This movement can cause back problems if you don't do it properly. You must lift the weight with the large muscles of your thighs and buttocks. It is in these muscles, and not the arms and shoulders, that the explosive power should originate.

### Seated Pulley Rowing

**Basic movement**: This exercise can be done on a machine specially designed for it or on the pulley station of a Universal Gym. Take a grip on the pulley handle or hand grips so that your hands are about six inches apart. Sit down and brace your feet against the foot bar at the base of the machine. Straighten your legs to take up the slack on the pulley and lean forward at about a 45-degree angle from the floor. Your arms should be straightened out so as to stretch the latissimus muscles. Simultaneously lean backwards until your back is perpendicular with the floor and bend your arms to bring the pulley handle toward your body until it touches the lower ribcage. Return the pulley bar to the starting position, resisting the pull of gravity, and repeat.

**What it does**: Pulley rowing is a movement similar to the bent barbell rowing exercise that you were introduced to in the beginning gym program. It works the latissimus dorsi muscles of the back, as well as the trapezius muscle of the upper back, the lower back, the biceps, and the forearms.

**Variations on a theme**: You can also do pulley rowing with the palms facing up instead of down on the handle or cable grips.

**Special considerations**: Since the latissimus muscles function by pulling the upper arms downward and back, emphasize this motion when doing the exercise. This is a general consideration when doing any exercise of this type. You want the movement to approximate as closely as possible the way the muscles are used in everyday or sports activities. Arch your back at the finish of each rep so that your lats are fully contracted and be sure to keep your elbows as close to the sides of your body as you can, so that the pulling motion is concentrated as much as possible in your back and not in your arms.

### Dumbbell Rows

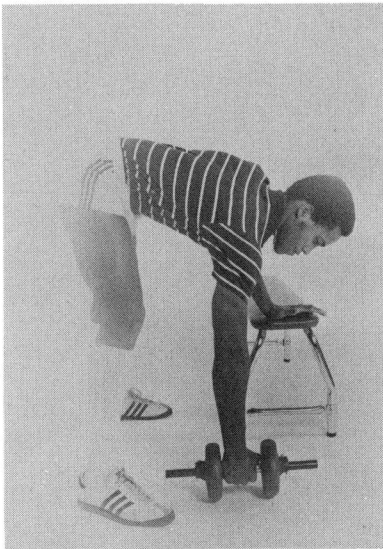

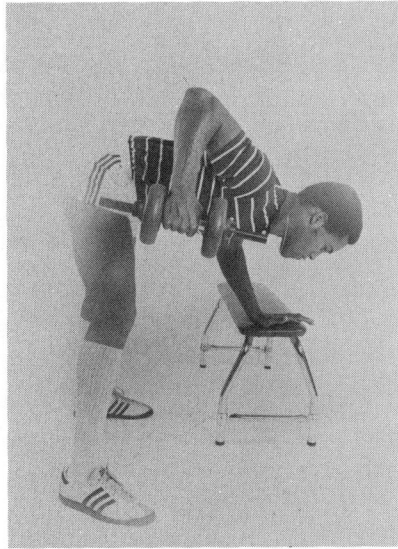

We introduced rowing motions with the barbell earlier in the basic program. Some people find that the exercise is more effective for them if they use a dumbbell instead. Grasp a dumbbell in one hand, bend forward at your waist, bracing yourself with your free hand on a convenient bench or post, and sequentially pull the dumbbell up to the side of your lower chest and lower it until your arm is fully extended. This is a great latissimus exercise, like all rowing motions, and you may find this an interesting change of pace from other rowing exercises. This movement works best if you alternate arms, doing a set with one arm and then with the other arm, so that each side has a brief rest before the next set.

**Dumbbell Rows**

Dumbbell rows can be done using a bench and a dumbbell. Begin with the weight on the floor and bring it up to your armpit.

**Hyperextensions**

**Basic movement**: This is another one of those exercises that uses a specialized piece of equipment, which not all gyms have. The movement is such a superior one though, especially after the difficult power exercises with the back muscles that I want to present it here. Get into the hyperextension bench, face down, hooking your heels under the smaller pad and supporting your hips by the larger pad so that your pelvis is just over the front edge of the larger pad. Put your hands behind your neck and interlock your fingers. Then allow your body to sag down until your torso is hanging straight down. The movement basically involves a reverse sit-up. Arch your back as high upward as you can in a smooth motion, i.e., without jerking. Return slowly to the starting position and repeat.

**What it does**: This is a fine stretching and conditioning exercise for the spinal erector muscles, with secondary emphasis on the buttocks, upper back and hamstrings.

**Variations on a theme**: More resistance, if you need it, can be added to this movement by holding a barbell plate behind your neck as you arch upward.

**Special considerations**: You may want to hold the stretch at the beginning of the movement when your torso is fully relaxed downward. You must make the upward arching motion a smooth one or you miss the purpose of the exercise and risk injury. If at any time you feel pain in this movement, discontinue it immediately. This exercise can bother the lower back, although most lifters experience beneficial loosening in the lower back following a few sets of slowly done hyperextensions.

**SHOULDER EXERCISES**
**Side Lateral Raises**

**Basic movement**:
**Dumbbells**: Stand erect with your feet shoulder-width apart and your toes pointed outward slightly. Holding a dumbbell in each hand so that the palms are facing each other as you hold the dumbbells in front of your thighs, lock your elbows and slowly raise your arms upward and to the sides until the dumbbells are raised to shoulder level. Slowly lower your arms back to the starting position and repeat.

## Side Lateral Raises

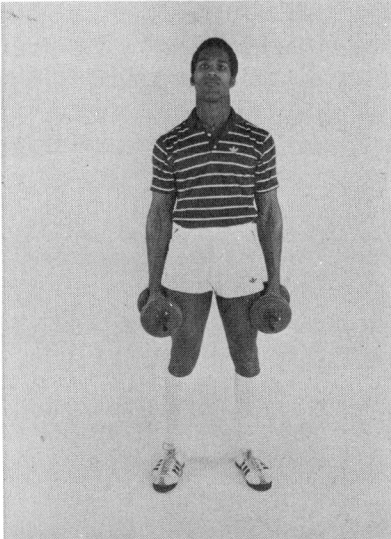

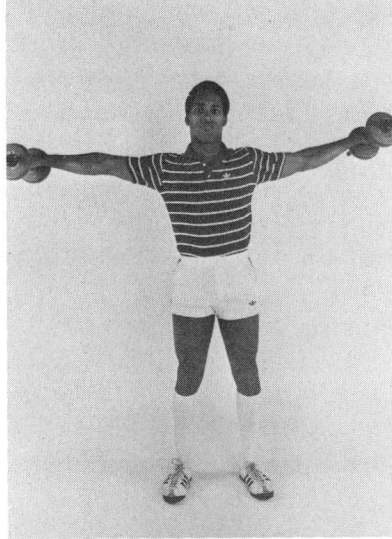

Begin side lateral raises with dumbbells at your side. Extend the arms and lock the elbows, with the dumbbells parallel to the floor.

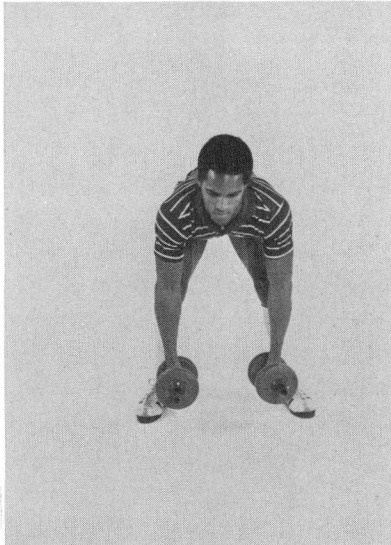

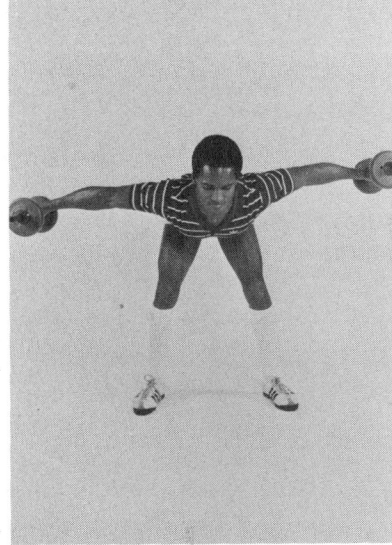

Side lateral raises can be done with your back bent. The motion and position is similar to bent rowing.

**What it does**: Lateral raises directly isolate the deltoid muscles.

**Nautilus**: Many sports conditioning gyms will have a Nautilus or similar machine to do side lateral raises on. Sit in the machine and adjust the seat height until the tops of your shoulders are approximately even with the pressing handles. You will be facing away from the weight stack, with the seat belt (if there is one) secured across your lap. Cross your ankles or otherwise keep your feet off the floor. With your palms facing each other and your hands open, slide the outsides of your lower forearms against the inner surface of the pads to either side. Grasp the handles attached to the pads and raise your arms straight out until your elbows are locked and your upper arms are slightly above an imaginary line extending from your shoulders. Lower your arms slowly and repeat.

**What it does**: Lateral raises in any form directly work the deltoids and are essential for shoulder development. In the Nautilus variation, the effect is concentrated exclusively on the medial head of the deltoids, a muscle that is comprised of three heads—medial, anterior, and posterior. The dumbbell variation, as with most free weight exercises, is much more ammenable to alterations in form that isolate the movement on other portions of the deltoid muscle. Dumbbell raises can be done to the front of your body, in which case the effect is concentrated in the anterior deltoid. You can also bend forward at your waist, raising the weights to the sides and back. The so-called *bent lateral raise* is the single most important exercise for the development of the posterior head of the deltoids, a beautiful, often neglected, muscle group. Another variation within the front, side, or bent lateral movement is the rotation of your palms from the facing-down position at the start of the movement to the palms-up position at the conclusion of the lifting phase of the movement, i.e., when your upper arms are just higher than shoulder level. As you rotate your wrist, you will note that the effort of the exercise shifts from the medial portion of the deltoids to the anterior deltoid. We will see this variation again later in the intermediate arm exercises, because it is fundamentally important to development of the arm muscles as well as the shoulders. Bend your arm slightly and rotate your wrist and hand outward. Note that as you do this, the biceps muscle contracts. It contracts because in addition to flexing the upper arm, the biceps also function in the rotation of the arm. Since this is the way the body works, it makes sense to train it that way. The rotation of the hand and wrist outward is called *supination*, while the rotation of hand and wrist inward is termed *pronation*. Pronation/supination variations in your shoulder lateral exercises will pay big dividends in developing the shoulder muscles in the manner in which they are used in everyday and sports activities.

**Variations on a theme**: Work these front, side, and bent variations of the lateral raise into your workout, perhaps by doing a set each workout, or by doing front raises one day, lateral raises the next, and so on. Also begin to use the supination movement in some of your sets, so that its added training benefits will begin to sculpt the shoulders. This is a good series of movements to develop body awareness as it pertains to isolated muscle groups.

## Upright Rowing

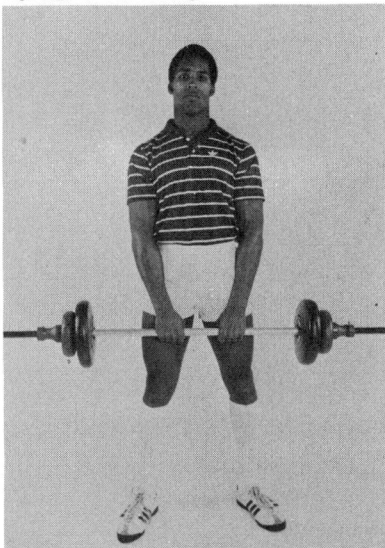

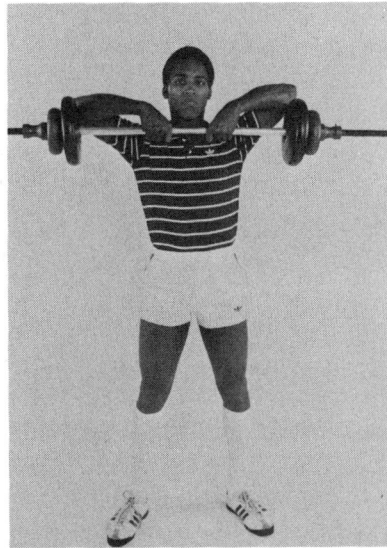

**Basic movement**: Stand erect with your feet placed shoulder-width apart and bend down and grasp a barbell with an overhand grip so that your palms are facing toward your legs, and your hands are only six to eight inches apart. Raise the bar to your thighs as if you were doing the power clean, i.e., lift with your legs and hips. Raise the bar from the front of your thighs up toward your chin by bending at your elbows and raising the weight with your shoulders and upper back. The movement is exactly as the name implies, a rowing movement done in the upright position. Lower the weight slowly to the starting position and repeat.

**Upright Rowing**

The upright row isolates the anterior deltoids. With the barbell at your waist, lift it as close to your chin as you can.

**What it does**: The upright row is the best isolation exercise for the anterior deltoids, with secondary emphasis on the trapezius muscles of the upper back.

**Variations on a theme**: The only real variation of this exercise, since it is already a highly isolationist movement to begin with, is to vary the distance between the hands. Most lifters find that a very narrow grip is most effective in stimulating the pump in the shoulders.

**Special considerations**: Try to lift the barbell as high as possible, right up to your chin. The movement should be fluid and unhurried, so that momentum does not play a part in either lifting the weight or lowering it. Keeping the barbell close to the body will isolate the movement more completely in the front of the shoulders.

## Shrugs

**Basic movement**: Grasp a dumbbell in each hand and allow your arms to hang free at your sides. With your arms in this position, shrug your shoulders upward, so that this movement raises the dumbbells without your arms moving (other than passively).

**Shrugs**

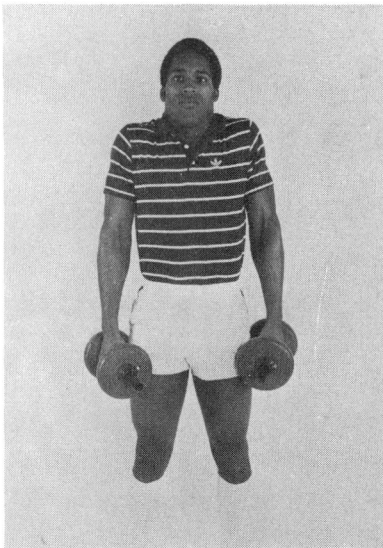

A good variation of shrugs is to rotate your shoulders slowly.

Slowly relax your shoulder and upper back muscles and return to the starting position.

**What it does**: The shrug is the best exercise to isolate the trapezius muscles at the upper portion of your back. The deltoids also receive secondary attention.

**Variations on a theme**: As you are doing shrugs, you can rotate your shoulders slowly by using a circular forward-and-back motion, so that all portions of the trapezius receive equal work.

**Special considerations**: Hold the fully shrugged position for a count or so at the top of the movement, so the trapezius is fully contracted.

## ARM EXERCISES
### Dumbbell Curls

**Basic movement**: There are many ways to do dumbbell curls, each of which stimulates the biceps muscles in different ways. We will cover some of the more important intermediate variations here, but keep in mind that you will undoubtedly see others in the literature or have them presented to you in the gym. The basic movement is similar to the barbell curl introduced in the basic programs. Grasp a dumbbell in each hand while standing erect. Your arms should be hanging down at your sides and your palms should be facing outward, thus gripping the dumbbell with an underhand grip. Pin your upper arms to your sides and curl the dumbbells upward in a semicircular movement to your chin. Lower the weights in the same arc and to the starting position and repeat. This movement can be done one hand at a time or with both hands simultaneously. The *restricted dumbbell incline curl* involves the same basic movement done on the incline bench or upright slant board. In this movement, your arms should be hanging down to the sides of the bench or slant board as you begin. Curl the weights upward in a fluid motion using only the power of your biceps. In *concentration curls*, sit on a flat bench, holding a dumbbell in one hand in an underhand grip, so that your elbow is resting on the inside of your leg for support. Bend forward at the waist, so that the dumbbell is extended toward the floor between your legs and your arm is straight. Curl the weight upward toward your chest, allowing only the forearm to move during the exercise. Lower the weight slowly and repeat.

**What it does**: All variations of dumbbell curls work the biceps

## Dumbbell Curls

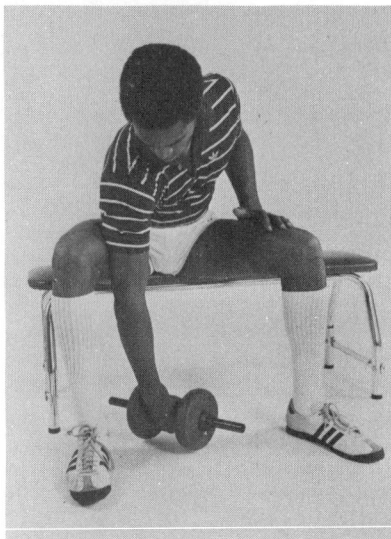

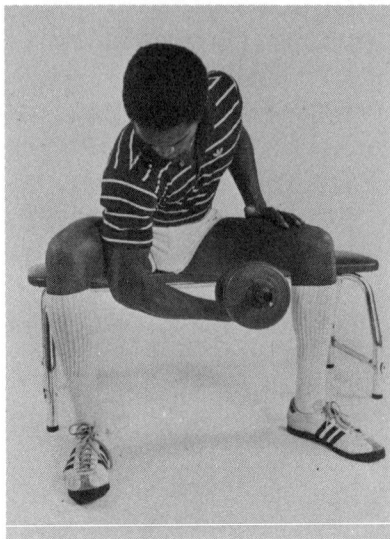

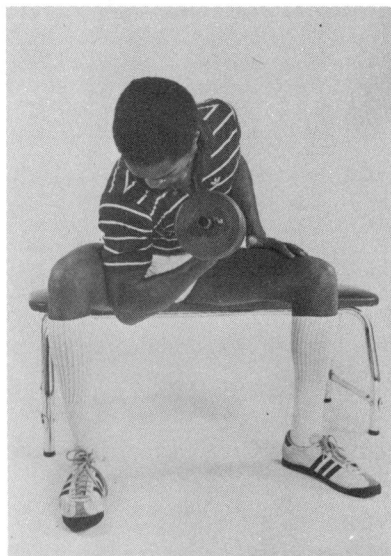

Concentration dumbbell curls include the bench. Curl the weight upward toward your chest. Rest your elbow on the inside of your leg for support.

## Dumbbell Curls (Cont.)

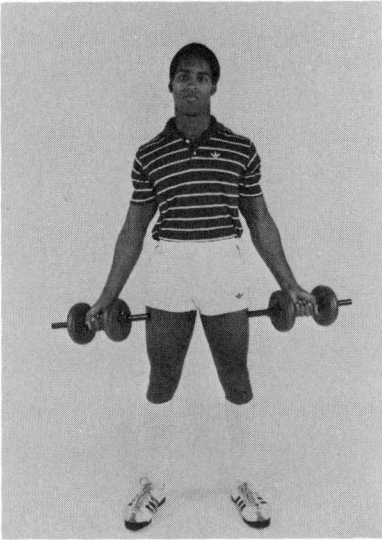

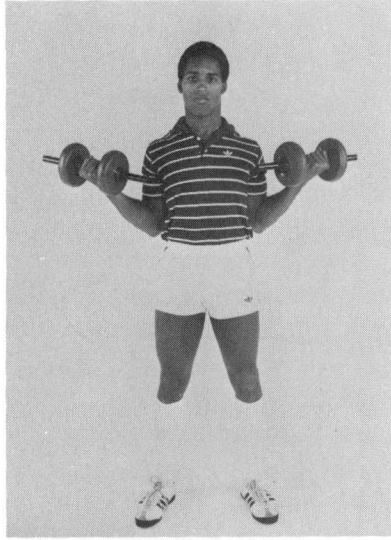

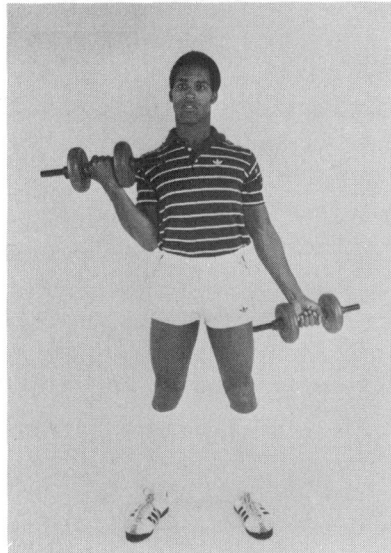

Dumbbell curls are similar to barbell curls. Curl the dumbbell to your chin during the upward movement. You can alternate arms during the exercise.

and brachialis muscles, with secondary emphasis on the forearms. These movements are highly effective in training the biceps because they isolate these muscles from other muscle groups, like the shoulders, which might tend to assist in the movement.

**Variations on a theme**: You should vary your workout to include at least two of these dumbbell exercises, because they attack the biceps in subtly different ways. The normal upright curl builds overall upper arm strength, while you will feel a superior stretching effect on the entire upper arm when doing the incline curl variation. Concentration curls are effective in developing the peak contraction component of upper arm flexion. Whichever of these variations you choose, remember to include supination of the wrists in all movements, so that the added training effect of twisting the arm will be noted. Simply rotate the wrists outward when curling the weight and rotate the wrists inward again when lowering them, and you will really feel the maximal contractive effort at the top of the movement. As in all exercises, particularly those involving the arms, make sure you isolate the effort in the arms. Do not allow momentum to enter into the movement or allow the shoulders to assist you.

**Special considerations**: As you become more proficient, you can introduce some isometric variations into these curling movements by holding the dumbbell stationary at various places in the exercise to stimulate peak contraction and facilitate total muscle fiber recruitment.

### Preacher or Scott Curls

**Basic movement**: This exercise was named after Larry Scott, the noted bodybuilder, and is perhaps the best isolation exercise for the biceps. It can be done using the preacher or Scott bench or on a Nautilus machine that approximates the same motion. The preacher bench is a small padded bench that rests on a metal pole. The pad is inclined at about a 45-degree angle and is positioned about three feet off the ground, or may be a special attachment to benches used for doing bench presses. The apparatus looks somewhat like a preacher pulpit, hence the name. Grasp a barbell using an underhand grip and either sit or stand behind the preacher bench, resting your upper arms on the padded support, so the arms are pointing downward and the barbell is held beyond the edge of the pad. Using only the power of your biceps, curl

## Scott Curls

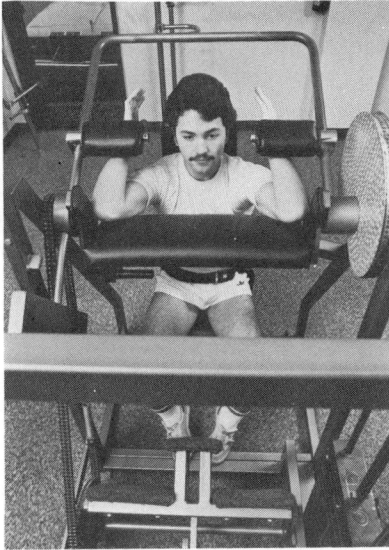

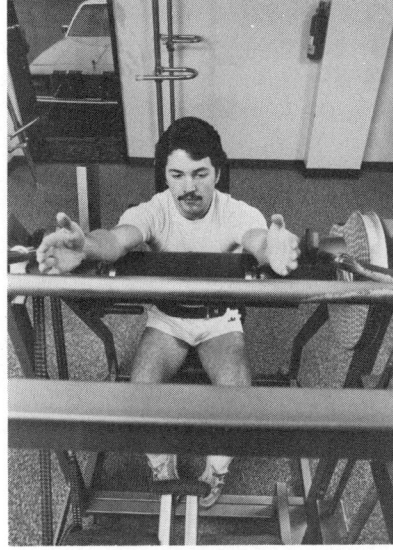

This Nautilus machine is similar to the Preacher Curls apparatus. The biceps and brachialis muscles are worked in this exercise.

the weight slowly upward to the level of the chin. Hold that position for a count or two, and slowly lower the weight to the starting position, repeating the movement as necessary. The Nautilus movement is similar, only you will be seated and raising a bar attached to a stack of weights with a cam system. Many gyms specializing in Nautilus machines may have several machines designed to do biceps curling motions. If you frequent such a gym, feel free to substitute these variations occasionally for free weight barbell or dumbbell exercises, but remember that you lose the added benefit of controlling the weights afforded by free weight variations.

**What it does**: Preacher curls are difficult exercises, designed to work the biceps and brachialis muscles. The movement, by design, is almost totally isolated in these muscles. The contraction afforded by preacher curls is maximal, but equally important, as you shall see when you do them, is the maximal stretch induced as you lower the weights. Remembering that the fitness of a muscle group is improved only by a combination of contraction and stretching motions, it is evident that the preacher curl makes a fine finishing exercise to the upper arm series.

**Variations on a theme**: As in all curling movements, you can vary the positions of your hands to alter the effects of the exercise. Placing your hands in a close grip, six inches or so apart, concentrates the effort in the outer biceps, while a wide, shoulder-width grip has proportionately greater effects on the inner biceps. You can also use supination in this movement, although your wrists are relatively fixed during the exercise. To stimulate the brachialis further, preacher curls can be done as you would do a reverse barbell curl. Grasp the barbell with an overhand grip, palms facing toward the floor.

**Special considerations**: Since this is a difficult exercise, the temptation to cheat on the movement may be great. Make sure the movement is slow and unhurried. Each complete rep should take nearly five seconds to complete. You may want to have a training partner handy, to assist you in completing those last few, difficult reps.

### Incline/Decline Triceps Extensions

Triceps extensions were covered in the basic program, but as an intermediate, you can begin adding another wrinkle to this valuable triceps exercise. Instead of doing extensions on a flat bench, do them either on an incline or decline bench. The effort will be much greater than that required on a flat bench, so have a spotter there to assist you if needed. You may also have a Nautilus triceps extension machine at your gym. If so, work Nautilus extensions into your program if you like, but be sure to include at least some free-weight sets into your routine.

### ABDOMINAL EXERCISES
### Twists/Side Bends

A variation of this exercise was introduced in the freehand program, but you may want to use it again in intermediate work. It is probably the best exercise around for the development of the obliques at the sides of the waist. Keeping your feet stationary, place a bar over your shoulders, grasping each end of it with your hands, and twist rapidly from side to side, moving only at your waist and hips.

With the exception of twists, the abdominal exercises introduced in the basic program are still the best movements you could do. Some exercises, as we have noted, are basic; you just can't get around them. Sit-ups, bent-leg raises, and the like, may not be especially interesting or fun to do, but they remain the basis of the abdominal program, regardless of your training proficiency.

## LEG EXERCISES

Again, the basic movements are still the best. You may find some specialized apparatus in your gym for doing calf raises or you may want to substitute leg presses occasionally for squats, but the squat, lunge, and calf raise are unique types of movements because they work the major muscle groups, but not at the expense of the detail work characteristic of the intermediate and advanced programs. You will simply add sets and resistance to these basic movements as you go along. You should especially concentrate on the lunge, because it is a fine movement for defining the thigh musculature. Leg extensions and leg curls, either on the Universal Gym or on a Nautilus machine, remain fine substitutes for the squat. The leg curl is especially valuable for the athlete needing both power and stamina in the hamstrings.

## INTERMEDIATE GYM ROUTINES

The intermediate routines presented here can act as a guide for your training. Keep in mind that we have noted throughout that several movements can be used interchangeably, especially when you have reached the intermediate training level. Your response to various exercises will be more apparent here than they were in the basic programs. You will need to experiment a bit now to find what works best for you. You should follow these programs with a nod to the various intermediate techniques presented at the beginning of this section. Keep in mind that your current level of fitness dictates that you vary your program fairly frequently and strive at all times for maximum effort in each set and movement. These programs can be adapted for split-routines or you can continue working out three days per week.

As in the basic programs, you will generally strive for 8 to 10 reps per set, doing three sets per movement, except in Nautilus exercises, where two sets will do. Individual considerations or time constraints may make it desirable for you to alter this strategy, using the rep and set variations described earlier in this section.

There really are no hard and fast rules to follow in this regard, because you must now become your own expert on the best way to train for your particular goals. The only constant is that each muscle group should be thoroughly exhausted at the conclusion of a series of sets designed to affect a particular body part.

### A Comprehensive Intermediate Program for Any Gym

Bench presses (Free weight or Universal)
Incline/decline presses (Free weight or Universal)
Dumbbell flies (Free weight; flat, incline, or decline bench)
Pullovers (Free weight or Nautilus)
Parallel bar dips (Free weight)
Power cleans (Free weight)
Bent barbell rowing (Free weight) *or*
Seated pulley rowing (Apparatus or Universal)
Hyperextensions (Free weight)
Lat machine pulldowns (Lat machine or Universal)
Chins (Chinning bar)
Military press (Free weight or Universal)
Upright rowing (Free weight) *or*
Dumbbell lateral raises (Free weight)
Shrugs (Free weight)
Barbell curls (Free weight)
Dumbbell curls (Free weight) *or*
Restricted incline dumbbell curls (Free weight)
Concentration curls (Free weight)
Preacher bench curls (Free weight or Nautilus)
Triceps extensions (Free weight or Nautilus; flat, incline, or
decline bench) *or*
French curls (Free weight)
Squats (Free weight) *or*
Lunges (Free weight) *or*
Leg presses (Free weight or Universal)
Leg curls (Free weight, Universal, Nautilus)
Calf raises (calf machine, free weight, or Universal)
Sit-ups (Free weight) *or*
Leg extensions/bent-leg raises (Free weight)

As you can see, the intermediate-level program is considerably more strenuous than the basic programs. You may not be able to do three sets of every movement in the beginning. In fact, it may well take the better part of a year to master this program. Start out by doing two good sets of every movement and work your way up. The exercises denoted as either/or alternatives may be substituted for each other whenever you like. The only exercise in which you should as a rule strive for high rep (i.e., 20 reps and up) sets, regardless of your goals, are the sit-ups or other abdominal exercises. Other than that, you can pick and choose parts of the above program, just as long as you include 8 to 10 sets per body part. For example, you might elect to do three sets of both incline and decline bench presses, followed by three sets of dumbbell flies, for your chest workout for a few weeks or so, and then change the workout slightly, so that you do two sets each of flat, incline, and decline bench presses, two sets of flies, and two sets of pullovers. Listen to what your body is telling you and alter your workout accordingly.

Remember to warm down after the workout and prior to hitting the sauna and shower. The intermediate workout, if done at a fairly rapid pace, will stimulate cardiovascular fitness. Nonetheless, most people interested in top overall conditioning will still want to run or swim on off-gym days. Just remember the cautions previously mentioned about the dangers of overtraining. It is far better to do fewer sets, making each set a *quality* set. In fact, many advanced gym athletes only do one or two sets of each exercise, preferring instead to work the muscle maximally on every rep.

After you have been on an intermediate training regimen for a few months, you will have achieved a fitness level truly uncommon in the American population. By any definition, you will be in better condition than 99 percent of the adult population, including those individuals already active in sports. You can maintain this fitness level as long as you stay on the intermediate program.

You will find that your progress occasionally plateaus. This is a time when no amount of work seems to facilitate further gains in fitness. During these periods, resist the temptation to work even harder unless you can avoid the danger of overtraining. Plateaus can usually be overcome by varying your routine slightly, thereby attacking the body from a different perspective and forcing renewed progress. The most important facet of intermediate and advanced gym training is that you must continually present the body and mind with new challenges. If you don't, you will begin to lose interest and your progress will flag. Many new perspectives on exercise are available in current periodicals and books on gym training. If you keep up with the literature, you will always find new and different exercises and techniques.

After several months or even up to a year on the intermediate program, you may want to move up to advanced training. Most advanced gym athletes are currently interested in bodybuilding per se, but increasing numbers of high-caliber athletes are seeing the rewards of advanced training in their own individual sports. The difference between intermediate and advanced training boils down to attitude. The advanced trainee is seeking not just a very high level of strength and fitness, but perfection. For this reason, you may not want to commit yourself to the time and work it takes to reach your potential. Nonetheless, advanced techniques can be used by the advanced intermediate as a change of pace.

# 7

# Advanced Gym Training

In advanced training you have learned enough about your own body and the way it works to be your own teacher. No one else knows as well as you do what your goals are and how your body responds to certain types of exercise and training techniques. Your body is now a responsive machine, capable of hard work and having endurance. When you evaluate your present competence in the four components of fitness, you see marked excellence across the board. You are lean, flexible, powerful, and aerobically fit. Still, the last month or two you do not seem to be making progress. Certain body parts or muscle groups apparently are lagging behind the others, no matter what you try. You are still interested in progress, but unsure how to go about it. First, you must reassess your individual goals and decide what you aspire to in your gym work. If you want more muscle mass, now is the time to begin going for it. If you want to keep your weight stable, but still desire increased power and athletic competence, certain advanced techniques can help you achieve this. At this stage of the game your progress will become increasingly a mental factor. The mind must either become your staunchest ally or you will find it difficult to move beyond the intermediate stage.

Advanced training is almost entirely technique-oriented. The exercises you will do are nearly the same as those of the intermediate program. What changes is the way the movements are done. The intensity level used in advanced techniques "tricks" the body into responding. Your body will be pushed into further progress by techniques that fire all your muscle fibers. The work is difficult and you should incorporate no more than one advanced technique in your program at once.

## ADVANCED TECHNIQUES

### Pre-exhaustion

Many of the basic exercises and, to a degree, the intermediate movements as well, work a large muscle group in combination with a smaller one. For example, the bench press is primarily a chest exercise, but triceps and deltoid strength are also important to the movement. The small muscles usually become fatigued before the large ones. In this manner your progress in the bench press may become limited by fatigue in the weaker deltoid muscles, and the pectorals may never be exercised enough to develop. Because these smaller, auxiliary muscles limit the full range of work of the larger ones, it is necessary to find a method of working the bigger muscle groups more thoroughly prior to doing the basic movements essential for development of the large functional muscle groups. Should your progress in basic exercises like the bench press or lat pulldowns become stuck, the use of pre-exhaustion techniques will usually restore progress.

Pre-exhaustion amounts to doing a set of isolation exercise for the larger muscle group and, with no rest, doing a basic movement for the same group. Recall that isolation exercises, such as those stressed in the intermediate programs, work a single muscle group, while the basic movements develop fitness in large, functionally related muscle groups. For example, dumbbell side lateral raises isolate the deltoid muscles, and flies isolate the pectorals. Similarly, the military press stimulates the triceps as well as the deltoids, while the bench press works the pectorals, deltoids, and triceps. Pre-exhaustion temporarily makes the larger muscle groups slightly weaker than the smaller groups, so that you can push the basic movement exceedingly hard.

Here are some examples of combinations of isolation exercises with basic movements. You can readily come up with others because of your experience, and this technique can be used on any muscle or muscle groups.

**Deltoids**: Dumbbell side lateral raises followed by military presses or seated presses.

**Pectorals**: Flies followed by bench presses or incline/decline presses.

**Latissimus dorsi**: Pullovers followed by bent rowing or lat machine pulldowns.

**Thighs**: Leg extensions followed by squats, lunges, or leg presses.

You can see that you were already incorporating a form of pre-exhaustion training in your intermediate program. Go from one set of isolation exercise to a set of the basic movement as rapidly as possible, because a rest period will defeat the purpose of the technique. Do no more than two sets, one isolation and one basic, in any given workout, although you can include as many of the muscle groups as you want in each workout.

**Forced Reps**: Generally, you finish a set by trying as hard as you can to get one last rep, and then terminate the movement. The problem with this approach is that your muscle is still not totally fatigued at this point; all of the muscle fibers have not been re-cruited into action. Using a training partner to assist you, you can do a few more reps than you could normally do alone. By taking a little bit more resistance off on each of the last several reps of a set, you can push yourself past the momentary point of failure in each exercise, thereby forcing the muscle to adapt. To experiment on forced rep methodology, try the bench press. Have your partner stand at the head of the bench. Do as many reps as you can without assistance and then try one more. As you begin to fail lifting the weight, your partner should grasp the middle of the bar and pull just hard enough to let you finish. Do two or three more such reps, with your partner assisting a bit more each time. The forced rep principle works for every exercise. Just be sure to use this variation only on the last set of your series of that particular exercise.

**Negative Reps**: This training variation is similar to forced reps. When your muscle is fatigued, you will not have enough power to raise the weight up, but you will still have enough energy to re-sist the pull of gravity as you lower the weight. When you can no longer force the weight upward, lower it slowly with assistance from your partner, and allow him to help you raise the weight. Then, as you lower the weight, your training partner pushes down-ward. The object is for you to resist this additional downward force as well as you can, allowing your partner to help you raise the weight, and repeating this process for three or four reps.

**Peaking and Tapering With Weights**: This advanced technique is especially valuable for the competitive athlete who is both train-ing in the gym and training for an individual sport. During the competitive season you should not work out in the gym more than two days per week, and in no case should one of those workout days be the day before a competition. The length of your competitive season will, of course, vary depending on your sport. Peaking during this competitive phase of the year simply involves pushing harder and harder until a week to ten days before competition. Gradually use heavier weights and perform movements faster and faster, including some of the other advanced training methods included in this section, timing your most intense workout of the season to fall seven to ten days before the most important early competition. After this point, taper off your gym workouts by doing three progressively lighter workouts at three- or four-day intervals. Start out the first tapering workout by using about 75 percent of the weight and sets you normally use. During the next workout, do a 50-50 combination, and if you do a third, drop down all the way to about 30-30. Try to do these sets as fast as you can, resting only 15 to 30 seconds between sets.

Tapering and peaking are difficult skills, as anyone presently involved in a competitive sport will attest. You will need to do some experimentation to find the progression that suits you best, but it is a skill well worth knowing and one that will give you the competitive edge.

**Supersets**: Supersets are variations of the pre-exhaustion technique previously described. Any series of exercises that work the same muscle or groups of muscles can be supersetted. The idea is to go from set to set, without a rest period between sets, starting from an isolation exercise and progressing to a basic movement. A superset may involve three or four exercises of one to three sets each. One example might be a chest superset starting with a set of dumbbell flies, then progressing through a set each of pullovers, incline bench presses, and flat bench presses. A thigh superset might start out with a set of leg extensions, followed by sets of squats and lunges, respectively. Supersets are extremely exhausting, so don't use them on every workout and don't superset more than one muscle group on any given workout day until you have adapted to the increased workload.

**High-Intensity Training**: This advanced technique is gaining increasing prominence among top-flight bodybuilders. It has a distinct advantage over many other advanced workout strategies in that a complete workout can be completed in about an hour, whereas most advanced routines may take over an hour and a half to complete. In high-intensity training, the muscle groups are worked almost continuously and nearly always to the point of exhaustion, never allowing the muscle group being worked to fully relax. Sets and reps are done more or less continuously, using moderately heavy weights and 6 to 8 reps per set. Some weight-lifters use very high set routines, with fairly light weights, often doing a series of five or more sets of the same movement and then five sets of another movement designed to work the same muscle or muscle group. As in supersetting, work into this routine gradually and never use high-intensity techniques all the time or on more than one muscle group at a time, or you seriously risk overtraining.

**Priority Techniques**: This is a simple variation that everyone can work into their training. We all have certain muscles or muscle groups that seem to lag behind the others in their development. These developmental imbalances should be corrected as soon as they are noted. Do this by working your lagging muscle group first in the workout, when your energy level is highest. You should also do more sets and put more intensity into your sets when dealing with the underdeveloped muscle group. By following your progress, you will readily be able to spot muscles that need priority treatment. The worst thing you can do is to continue to favor your strong points and gloss over your weaknesses. There is a strong temptation to do this, particularly if your strong points are highly visible and your weak areas are hidden. This is one of the reasons we stressed the importance of honest self-evaluation earlier and why it is important to work out in relatively brief attire and in front of mirrors. The weak areas will continue to fall farther and farther behind if left without attention and soon you will begin to develop in a visibly non-symmetric fashion. Nothing looks worse than a set of bulging biceps sitting on underdeveloped shoulders or triceps. Remember, the sole purpose of developing the body in the gym is to produce a symmetrical, totally fit body.

Individual progress beyond the intermediate stage can only be forecast in generalities. You will get stronger and fitter as you continue to work out, but at this stage, genetic potential casts its shadow over the picture. Each of you has an innate capacity for muscular size and strength, and as you approach this limit your progress will slow. The innate capacity is almost never reached in most of us, however, so you should not feel limited in any way.

## THE ADVANCED GYM PROGRAM

Each of you will have differing goals for your continued progress in the gym. For this reason, and because there are literally hundreds of possible exercises that you could be doing at this stage of the game, the best sample program for your advanced training would be one similar to that which you used as an intermediate. As an advanced trainee, you should build on that program, adding new exercises every few weeks from among those that were presented in this book and in other sources, especially those particularly good references listed in the appendix. You should also begin experimenting with some of the advanced training techniques presented in this chapter. You will find now that your progress is directly related to *how* you do the exercises and not so much as to which ones you do. But follow this general rule: Most experts agree that any advanced program should include at least nine or so sets per body part (i.e., the chest, the back, the biceps, the deltoids, etc.) unless you are supersetting or using some other particular variation for that set of muscles. You may see more plateaus in the advanced level than you encountered before, but work past these by altering your routine and getting out of the rut every so often. You must pay close attention to your diet and sleep habits. In addition, the advanced trainee must especially keep in mind the admonition that the mind and body be hungry for more at all times. This will be increasingly difficult as the months turn into years and after you reach the state at which you feel satisfied with your level of achievement. Nonetheless, fatigue brought on by too much training or by staleness can easily lead to overtraining. Should you find that you have become overtrained, lay off for a week or so until your enthusiasm returns.

Most people will find that the split routine training schedule works best for them when trying to play their advanced training battle plan. Your participation in other sports will have a large bearing on how often or on what days of the week you should or can train. Whatever routine you decide on, make sure it includes adequate time for warm-up and warm-down activities and for at least some running, swimming, or other aerobic activities.

The following chapter is designed specifically for athletes in various sports who have reached the advanced level in the gym and want to tailor their advanced training to their particular sport. Perhaps you never envisioned yourself as a serious athlete before, but now you should see endless possibilities in your sport.

# 8

# Individualized Gym Programs for Various Sports

As an advanced gym athlete you can opt for one of three approaches in continuing your training. You can continue to add difficulty to the gym training program and attempt to join the ranks of elite bodybuilders, in the broadest sense of the word. Alternately, you may want to begin specializing your training more in accord with the demands of specific sports. Of course, the third alternative would be to try to maintain your good condition for the rest of your life.

This chapter is designed to help those of you interested in the second alternative—the application of gym training, at the advanced level, to sports programs. The programs presented here are applicable to a number of gym situations and are equally useful for male or female athletes. All are for the off-season in your competitive schedule. They should be used with the considerations presented in Chapter 7 on peaking and tapering with weights during the competitive season, to form the basis for a sports-efficient gym training program.

Each of the following programs is designed with the advanced trainee in mind, so the beginner or intermediate who might want to begin using them should cut the number of sets back to his ability level. Serious athletes can use these programs as a basis to evolve their own individual gym training programs. As we have seen, the advanced athlete must take charge of his own training schedule for maximal progress.

## THE CORE MODULE OF EXERCISES

Regardless of your particular sport, there is a module of basic exercises that comprehensively work the major muscle groups and that are essential to your progress. The additional exercises will zero in on the specific muscles important in each sport discussed. The basic module consists of the following exercises:

| Exercise | Sets | Rep Range |
|---|---|---|
| Bench Press | 3 | 10-15 |
| Lat Machine Pulldowns or Bent Rowing | 3 | 8-12 |
| Military Press | 3 | 8-12 |
| Upright Curls | 3 | 8-12 |
| Squats/Lunges | 3 | 10-12 |
| Calf Raises | 3 | 15-20 |
| Sit-Ups/Leg Raises | 3 | 30+ |

The module itself would make a fine program for most athletes and would result in improved sports performance, but the following movements will foster tremendous gains in athletic competence. You should do the module exercises prior to the individual exercises specific to each sport. It goes without saying that this workout, like all others, should be preceded with a warmup and followed with a warmdown. You can use either the split-routine training method or train three times per week.

## INDIVIDUAL SPORTS PROGRAMS

### Alpine Skiing

All forms of downhill skiing demand strength in the quadriceps muscles of the thigh and the trunk stabilizing muscles, especially the abdominals and the lower back. To foster this strength, do the core program and the following exercises:

| Exercise | Sets | Rep Range |
|---|---|---|
| Sit-Ups | 2 | 50+ |
| Hyperextensions | 2 | 15-20 |
| Leg Extensions | 3 | 15-20 |
| Leg Curls | 3 | 15-20 |
| Leg Presses | 3 | 15-20 |

### Badminton/Tennis

These sports use leg strength for stopping and starting as well as upper body strength, especially in the deltoids and forearms.

| Exercise | Sets | Rep Range |
|---|---|---|
| Hyperextensions | 1 | 10-15 |
| Side Lateral Raises | 3 | 10-15 |
| Upright Rowing | 3 | 10-15 |
| Lat Machine Pushdowns *or* French Curls | 3 | 10-15 |
| Barbell Curls | 3 | 10-15 |
| Reverse Curls | 3 | 10-15 |
| Leg Press | 3 | 20-30 |
| Leg Curl | 3 | 20-30 |
| Calf Machine | 3 | 20-30 |
| Twists | 1 | 50+ |

## Baseball

Baseball is a sport requiring general body strength, especially in the legs, deltoids and arms.

| Exercise | Sets | Rep Range |
|---|---|---|
| Parallel Bar Dips | 3 | 10-12 |
| Chins | 3 | 8-12 |
| Bent Lateral Raises | 3 | 8-12 |
| Triceps Extensions | 3 | 8-12 |
| Lunges | 2 | 15-20 |
| Calf Machine | 3 | 20-30 |

## Basketball

The excellent basketball player is skilled at jumping and running, and also has the upper body strength to play a physical game under the boards.

| Exercise | Sets | Rep Range |
|---|---|---|
| Dumbbell Lateral Raises | 3 | 10-12 |
| Triceps Extensions | 3 | 8-12 |
| Pullovers | 3 | 8-12 |
| Deadlifts | 1 | 10-15 |
| Leg Extensions | 3 | 15-20 |
| Leg Curls | 3 | 15-20 |
| Seated Calf Machine | 2 | 20-30 |

### Bicycling

The bicyclist is interested in leg strength, but upper body power and stamina also come into play.

| Exercise | Sets | Rep Range |
|---|---|---|
| Crunches/Leg Extensions | 3 | 30+ |
| Leg Extensions | 5 | 10-15 |
| Leg Curls | 5 | 10-15 |
| Lunges | 3 | 10-15 |
| Calf Machine | 3 | 20-30 |

### Boxing

The punching power of the boxer comes from the deltoids, pectorals, and triceps. Lower body stamina, especially in the calves, is also important.

| Exercise | Sets | Rep Range |
|---|---|---|
| Incline Press | 3 | 6-8 |
| Decline Press | 3 | 6-8 |
| Flies | 3 | 10-12 |
| Parallel Bar Dips | 3 | 10-12 |
| Chins | 2 | 10-12 |
| Side Lateral Raises | 3 | 10-15 |
| Dumbbell Curls | 3 | 10-15 |
| Lat Machine Pushdowns | 3 | 10-12 |
| Reverse Curls | 3 | 10-12 |
| Hyperextensions | 2 | 15-20 |
| Crunches | 2 | 30+ |
| Calf Raises | 3 | 30+ |

### Canoeing

In canoeing, the shoulders, back, and arms undergo considerable stress, as do the abdominals.

| Exercise | Sets | Rep Range |
|---|---|---|
| Pullovers | 4 | 10-15 |
| Bent Rowing *or* Pulley Rowing | 3 | 10-12 |
| Side Lateral Riases | 3 | 10-15 |
| Bent Lateral Raises | 3 | 10-15 |
| Parallel Bar Dips | 2 | 10-15 |

| | | |
|---|---|---|
| Dumbbell Curls | 3 | 8-12 |
| Sit-Ups/Crunches | 3 | 30+ |

### Climbing
The rock climber needs balanced, overall strength.

| Exercise | Sets | Rep Range |
|---|---|---|
| Incline Press | 3 | 6-10 |
| Parallel Bar Dips | 3 | 8-12 |
| Chins | 3 | 8-12 |
| Pulley Rowing | 3 | 10-15 |
| Dumbbell Lateral Raises | 3 | 8-12 |
| Bent Lateral Raises | 3 | 8-12 |
| Dumbbell Curls | 3 | 8-12 |
| French Curls *or* Triceps Extensions | 3 | 8-12 |
| Leg Extensions | 3 | 10-15 |
| Leg Curls | 3 | 10-15 |
| Lunges | 3 | 10-15 |

### Football
Different positions in football require various bodily attributes, but all positions require superior overall strength and explosive power, with particular emphasis on the pushing muscles.

| Exercise | Sets | Rep Range |
|---|---|---|
| Incline Press | 3 | 8-12 |
| Decline Press | 3 | 8-12 |
| Flies | 3 | 8-12 |
| Pullovers | 3 | 8-12 |
| Parallel Bar Dips | 3 | 8-12 |
| Deadlifts | 3 | 10-15 |
| Seated Press | 3 | 8-12 |
| Upright Rowing | 4 | 10-15 |
| Leg Extensions | 3 | 15-20 |
| Leg Curls | 3 | 15-20 |
| Shrugs | 3 | 10-15 |
| Triceps Extensions | 3 | 8-12 |
| Calf Machine Raises | 4 | 15-20 |
| Sit-Ups | 2 | 30+ |

Note: You can vary the order of these exercises as you wish.

## Golf

You usually don't associate strength with golf, but some of the best golfers on the pro tour are finding that gymwork helps their game tremendously. The emphasis is on the deltoids and arms, but since the golf swing integrates the whole body, the basic module followed by the following movements will really improve your power.

| Exercise | Sets | Rep Range |
| --- | --- | --- |
| Bent Lateral Raises | 3 | 10-15 |
| Side Lateral Raises | 3 | 10-15 |
| Reverse Curls | 3 | 10-15 |
| Dumbbell Curls | 3 | 10-15 |
| Lat Machine Pushdowns | 3 | 10-15 |

## Gymnastics

The gymnast in particular will note the effects of having one muscle or muscle group that is weaker than the others. With the help of your coach, identify these muscles and select one or two exercises from the preceding sections; they are designed to isolate them. Do three to five sets of these movements after completing the basic module.

## Handball/Racquetball

The handball/racquetball player needs the same basic power/ speed attributes as the tennis player.

| Exercise | Sets | Rep Range |
| --- | --- | --- |
| Flies | 2 | 8-12 |
| Parallel Bar Dips | 1 | 8-12 |
| Side Lateral Raises | 2 | 10-15 |
| Bent Lateral Raises | 2 | 10-15 |
| Lat Machine Pushdowns *or* | 2 | 10-15 |
| Triceps Extensions | 2 | 10-15 |
| Twists | 2 | 30+ |
| Sit-Ups | 2 | 30+ |
| Hyperextensions | 1 | 10-15 |
| Leg Extensions | 2 | 15-20 |
| Lunges | 2 | 15-20 |
| Calf Machine Raises | 2 | 20-30 |

**Hockey** (Ice or Field)

Top-flight hockey players have exceptional leg and deltoid strength, as well as well-developed arms, chests, abdominals, and lower back muscles. To attain balanced skating power as well as the ability to slap in a goal, do the basic module and the following exercises.

| Exercise | Sets | Rep Range |
| --- | --- | --- |
| Dumbbell Flies | 2 | 10-15 |
| Incline Presses | 2 | 10-15 |
| Decline Presses | 2 | 10-15 |
| Parallel Bar Dips | 2 | 8-12 |
| Dumbbell Side Laterals | 3 | 10-15 |
| Bent Lateral Raises | 3 | 10-15 |
| Triceps Extensions | 3 | 10-15 |
| Dumbbell Curls | 3 | 8-12 |
| Reverse Curls | 3 | 8-12 |
| Sit-Ups | 2 | 30+ |
| Twists | 2 | 30+ |
| Leg Extensions | 4 | 15-20 |
| Leg Curls | 4 | 15-20 |

**Karate/Kung Fu/Judo**

The martial arts require both upper and lower body strength and quickness. The emphasis is on the pushing muscles of the upper body, especially the chest, shoulders, and triceps.

| Exercise | Sets | Rep Range |
| --- | --- | --- |
| Incline Press | 2 | 10-15 |
| Parallel Bar Dips | 2 | 8-12 |
| Chins | 2 | 8-12 |
| Seated Pulley Rowing | 2 | 10-15 |
| Side Lateral Raises | 3 | 10-15 |
| Bent Lateral Raises | 3 | 10-15 |
| Dumbbell Curls | 2 | 10-15 |
| Triceps Extensions *or* French Curls | 3 | 10-15 |
| Twists | 2 | 30+ |
| Crunches | 2 | 30+ |
| Lunges | 2 | 10-15 |
| Calf Machine Raises | 3 | 20-30 |

### Nordic Skiing

Cross-country skiing is an endurance sport that demands both leg power and pulling power in the upper body. Thus the specified workout concentrates on leg work and on developing the pulling muscles of the trunk.

| Exercise | Sets | Rep Range |
|---|---|---|
| Parallel Bar Dips | 3 | 8-12 |
| Pullovers | 3 | 10-15 |
| Pulley Rowing *or* | 3 | 10-15 |
| Dumbbell Rowing | 3 | 10-15 |
| Lat Machine Pushdowns | 3 | 10-15 |
| Reverse Curls | 3 | 10-15 |
| Leg Raises | 2 | 20-30 |
| Leg Extensions | 3 | 20-30 |
| Leg Curls | 3 | 20-30 |
| Seated Calf Machine | 3 | 20-30 |
| Lunges | 1 | 15-20 |

### Rugby

Although the rules of the game are different, rugby uses the same muscular skills as our professional football. To develop the power and speed necessary to excel at this grueling game, follow the same workout as that given for football, adding a set or two of hyperextensions in the 10-15 rep range.

### Running (Distance)

The distance runner needs the strength in leg, shoulder, arm, and back muscles to keep these groups from cramping and tiring during a long race. For this reason, all supplementary exercises are done in high-rep, low-set formats.

| Exercise | Sets | Rep Range |
|---|---|---|
| Bench Press | 2 | 20-30 |
| Parallel Bar Dips | 1 | 10-15 |
| Chins | 1 | 10-15 |
| Upright Rowing | 2 | 20-30 |
| Lat Machine Pulldowns | 1 | 20-30 |
| Dumbbell Curls | 1 | 20-30 |
| Deadlifts | 1 | 20-30 |
| Leg Raises | 1 | 30+ |

## Running (Middle-Distance)

The middle-distance events require stamina and speed in equal measure. Upper body power is especially important for the drive to the finish. To attain this power balance, follow the same routine given for long-distance running, adding two sets of deadlifts, in the range of 10-15 reps each.

## Running (Sprinting)

The sprinter depends on explosive leg power and upper body drive to excel.

| Exercise | Sets | Rep Range |
|---|---|---|
| Leg Press | 4 | 15-20 |
| Leg Curl | 4 | 15-20 |
| Lunges | 4 | 15-20 |
| Calf Press | 5 | 20-30 |
| Side Lateral Raises | 3 | 15-20 |
| Hyperextensions | 3 | 10-15 |
| Sit-Ups | 3 | 30+ |

## Skating (Ice or Roller)

Skaters need thigh and calf strength, with additional strength in the arms and shoulders.

| Exercise | Sets | Rep Range |
|---|---|---|
| Leg Extensions | 3 | 15-20 |
| Leg Curls | 3 | 15-20 |
| Calf Raises | 3 | 15-20 |
| Hyperextensions | 1 | 15-20 |
| Twists | 2 | 30+ |
| Sit-Ups | 2 | 30+ |

Note: Speed skaters should also include two sets of heavy squats or lunges in their program, in a range of 8-12 reps per set. Skaters who employ frequent lifting in their performances should also do two sets of heavy military presses in the range of 10-15 reps each.

### Swimming

Swimming uses all of the body musculature, with particular emphasis on the pulling muscles of the torso and arms.

| Exercises | Sets | Rep Range |
|---|---|---|
| Pullovers | 3 | 15-20 |
| Parallel Bar Dips | 3 | 10-15 |
| Chins | 3 | 10-15 |
| Seated Pulley Rowing | 3 | 15-20 |
| Triceps Extensions | 3 | 15-20 |
| Hyperextensions | 3 | 15-20 |
| Twists | 3 | 30+ |
| Sit-Ups | 3 | 30+ |
| Leg Extensions | 3 | 15-20 |
| Leg Curls | 3 | 15-20 |
| Calf Machine Raises | 3 | 20-30 |
| Lunges | 3 | 15-20 |

### Track and Field (Throwing Events)

Throwing events require explosive body strength, with emphasis on the chest, shoulders, and triceps. Leg power should not be neglected either, because throwing requires inputs from all of the body muscles, not just the trunk and arms.

| Exercise | Sets | Rep Range |
|---|---|---|
| Incline Press | 3 | 6-10 |
| Flies | 3 | 8-12 |
| Pullovers | 3 | 8-12 |
| Parallel Bar Dips | 3 | 10-15 |
| Chins | 3 | 10-15 |
| Hyperextensions | 2 | 10-15 |
| Military Press | 3 | 8-12 |
| French Curls | 3 | 8-12 |
| Triceps Extensions | 3 | 8-12 |
| Dumbbell Curls | 3 | 8-12 |
| Reverse Curls | 4 | 8-12 |
| Sit-Ups | 3 | 30+ |
| Twists | 3 | 30+ |
| Lunges | 3 | 10-15 |
| Leg Extensions | 3 | 10-15 |
| Leg Curls | 3 | 10-15 |

### Track and Field (Decathlon/Pentathlon)

The decathlon and pentathlon are by definition events that require an enormous amount of fitness in all of the body muscles. Your workout after the basic module should be somewhat similar to that described for the athletes in throwing events. However, you will want to use lighter weights and do more reps in each set. For example, do 10-15 reps in the military press instead of 8-12. In addition, substitute upright rowing for French curls, and add two or three sets of pulley rowing to the throwing workout. Feel free to mix this program up a bit to work those muscles that seem to impede your progress in certain events.

### Volleyball

The good volleyball player has the ability to jump vertically as well as the power to spike the ball and block shots. Spiking and blocking involve the throwing muscles.

| Exercise | Sets | Rep Range |
|---|---|---|
| Pullovers | 3 | 15-20 |
| Hyperextensions | 3 | 10-15 |
| Side Lateral Raises | 3 | 10-15 |
| Twists | 3 | 30+ |
| Leg Press | 4 | 15-20 |
| Calf Press | 4 | 15-20 |

### Wrestling

Wrestling is a sport requiring strength and stamina in all of the body muscles, but particularly in the pulling muscles of the upper body.

| Exercise | Sets | Rep Range |
|---|---|---|
| Parallel Bar Dips | 4 | 10-15 |
| Chins | 4 | 10-15 |
| Pullovers | 3 | 10-15 |
| Pulley Rowing | 3 | 10-15 |
| Military Press | 3 | 8-12 |
| Dumbbell Curls | 3 | 10-15 |
| Reverse Curls | 3 | 10-15 |
| Lunges | 3 | 10-15 |
| Hyperextensions | 2 | 10-15 |
| Upright Rowing | 3 | 15-20 |

| | | |
|---|---|---|
| Twists | 2 | 30+ |
| Crunches | 3 | 30+ |
| Leg Curls | 3 | 15-20 |

### Dedication vs. Fanaticism

The programs presented here and, in fact, any advanced-level training are tough and require a high degree of motivation to tackle. By the time you are an advanced gym athlete, you will be spending considerable time each week in the gym. If you are like most people, the further you go in your training the more you feel you can accomplish. The athlete who vigorously pursues excellence readily becomes addicted to his sport. The training regimen can become a compulsion and thus presents dangers to watch for. Deep psychological problems might even occur if injury or other circumstances force you to cease training, even if only for a brief period of time. Psychologists are becoming increasingly aware of the fact that addictions occur in normally beneficial activities as well as harmful habits. The athlete can become so addicted to his sport that family, job, and other important parts of life are left by the wayside.

As you continue along the road to whatever goals you have set for yourself, keep your training in perspective. Do not lose sight of the fact that we cannot all become Olympic-caliber athletes nor should most of us even try. Train for *yourself* and not for someone else. Enjoy and revel in the progress you have made and do not set unreasonable standards for achievement. Your fitness should be a source of pleasure to you, but if you become a fanatic, all pleasure will go out of your training. Your greatest enemy will inevitably become overtraining, and the effects of overtraining always result from continual overloads placed on your body as you are driven to success. Train for health, for fitness, and to look good, but never train out of compulsion.

# 9

# Nutrition for the Gym Athlete

Perhaps no aspect of athletic training causes more confusion or is fraught with more misinformation than the subject of proper nutrition. We are constantly bombarded with newspaper ads, television commercials and other media either showing us a new gadget to help us lose weight or touting some miracle food supplement. The health and fitness literature is loaded with ways to spend your hard-earned dollars pursuing the ideal training diet. The fact is, the ideal training diet is no diet at all, just the same sensible nutritional regimen your mother or grandmother impressed on you in your youth. There are no miracles, no shortcuts when it comes to fueling your body, only common sense and a nod to some basic nutritional principles. The old adage, "You are what you eat," is generally true. A bad nutritional strategy will undermine your progress as an athlete. The actual dietary regimen you elect to follow will be determined in part by your nutritional goals, i.e., whether you need to lose or gain weight. Nonetheless, there are certain constants in nutritional policy that are important to everyone, regardless of sex, age or fitness level.

## THE IDEAL TRAINING DIET

Regardless of what you might have read or heard, there are no magic foods nor any taboo foods in the ideal training diet. In fact, it is best to throw the very idea of "diet" out the window. The word diet may imply some special short-term regimen, usually extreme in nature, designed to rid the body of fat. What most diets do is provide, at best, short-term weight loss, generally comprised of water and lean body tissue as well as fat, which is quickly replaced as soon as the diet is terminated. Additionally, less than 10 percent of the reducing dieters who actually lose weight are able to keep that weight off for more than a few months. The only way to produce fundamental, long-term changes in your body composition is to combine a sound exercise program with a sensible eating plan. The exercise part of the formula has been discussed in this book. Now for the sound nutritional program.

The human body is an amazing carbon-based mechanism, capable of assimilating relatively simple carbon-based foods and assembling them into new tissue and the high-energy compounds necessary to run our machinery. Food's high-energy compounds are comprised of varying quantities of protein, carbohydrate, and fat, with tiny amounts of trace elements and minerals. Carbohydrates and fats function as energy-yielding molecules in the human body and there is no dietary requirement for these compounds, save for caloric needs themselves. Aside from certain unsaturated fatty acids, which are absolutely required by the body, the sole function of fats and carbohydrates is to provide energy. Protein on the other hand, is the key substance that builds muscle and must be consumed daily by the athlete. However, the dietary requirements for protein are rather minimal. Most of us eat far more protein than we need, and the excess is merely converted to other compounds and used for energy production or stored as fat. The adult male needs about 50 to 70 grams of protein each day to replace those amino acids, the components of protein molecules, that are broken down and turned over by the body on a daily basis. Women generally need even less, because their lean body weight is slightly less than men's. While a pregnant or lactating female may need about 70 or 80 grams of protein per day, the average female needs only 40 or 50 grams daily. This is only about two ounces, or as much protein supplied by two glasses of milk and a three-ounce portion of lean meat. Does the weight-training athlete require more protein than the sedentary individual? The most recent physiological evidence suggests that he does not. As you train, your body becomes more conservative in the turnover of its protein stores represented by muscle and organ tissues. Even very hard training will result in muscle mass gains or at best around 8 to 10 pounds per year, or just a few ounces per week. The best policy for the gym athlete is to plan a diet that supplies between 80 and 100 grams of protein per day. You probably eat much more than this now, so this should be no problem. Why not buy some insurance and eat much more than 100 grams per day just to be sure? Because excess protein in your diet places a greater load on many of your vital organs, especially your kidneys.

Because you are training, your need for calories will be higher than that of you sedentary friends. Get these calories not from rich, fatty foods, but from foods high in complex carbohydrates. Whole-grain bread, potatoes, and other foods high in starch contain many complex carbohydrates, which are digested slowly by your body, thus producing a constant trickle of blood sugar for your energy needs. Refined carbohydrates, like sugar, and yes, even honey, require no digestive process, and instead flood into the bloodstream almost immediately after consumption. Excess blood sugar is quickly drawn from your bloodstream and converted to fat. Constantly eating foods high in simple sugar leads directly to obesity. This is not to say that sweet foods must be struck off your training diet, but do use moderation.

What about fats and cholesterol? The role of high-fat diets in the development of heart and artery disease is currently a matter of controversy. Cholesterol is a compound produced in the body and required for the synthesis of many important metabolic substances. No one is sure about the role played by cholesterol consumed in the diet. Because of these controversies, it would be best to err on the side of safety and limit foods like fatty meats, eggs and whole milk, which are high in cholesterol. Most of us consume about 40 percent of our calories in the form of fat, since fat has about twice the calories per unit weight of either carbohydrates or protein. This figure should be cut to about 20 percent. The best training regimen is thus the best overall eating plan for all of us, and not a diet as such.

Plan for 15-20 percent of your calories to come from protien and about the same quantity for fats of all kinds. The rest of your caloric needs can come largely from complex carbohydrates.

How many calories do you need each day? It depends on the individual. In general, the moderately active male requires about 2500 calories per day for a body weight of about 160 pounds. At 200 pounds you might need about 2800 calories. A male in a very demanding, physical job might require 3500 to 4000 calories per day. An active female generally burns about 2000 to 2200 calories per day, more if she is heavy and less if she is small.

To this general rate is superimposed the 400 or so extra calories you burn in a typical workout. There is evidence that your basal metabolic rate, that is, the amount of energy required just to stay alive, remains elevated for several hours after you engage in heavy training, so that a few hundred extra calories will be consumed after a workout.

The only way to tell approximately how many calories you use every day is to monitor each and every bit of food you eat during a time when your weight is stable. This caloric value is a good estimate of your normal metabolic rate. You will find that this value decreases as you get older; at 55 only about 80 percent of the calories you needed at age 25 are burned. This is one of the reasons you gain weight a little at a time during adulthood. The average female will also gain about 20 pounds, nearly all of it as fat, between the age of 25 and 55. The average man adds about 15 pounds in the same time.

## LOSING FAT WHILE GAINING MUSCLE– THE KEY TO MUSCULAR DEFINITION

The only way to lose fat effectively is to lose it gradually by decreasing your caloric intake to a value slightly below the amount burned by the body. Those extra calories your body requires must then come from stored fat. You should not try to lose more than a pound or two per week. While faster weight losses are certainly possible, they will almost always come at the expense of lean body tissue and water. To lose one pound of fat per week, you need only restrict your caloric intake to a value 500 calories less than you burn up. It is easiest to accomplish this reduction by reducing fat intake, since each gram of fat has about 9 calories, while carbohydrates and protein contain only about 4.5 calories per gram. Losing two pounds per week requires a caloric deficiency of about 1000 calories per day, since one pound of fat comprises about 3500 calories.

Fad diets don't work and are potentially detrimental to your progress in the gym. Crash diets containing less than about 1200 calories per day simply cannot provide you with the protein, complex carbohydrates, vitamins, and minerals you need. Much of the weight you lose will be from muscle tissue and even vital organs. Low-carbohydrate diets are unadvisable for another reason. Carbohydrates are essential for the strength needed in the workout.

Your body is very inefficient at burning fat rapidly, as would be the case in a gym workout, and runs almost exclusively on muscle and liver glycogen, a form of stored starch. In addition, your brain must metabolize carbohydrate compounds, because it lacks the enzymes required for fat utilization. The low-carb diet will get the weight off, but also tire you so badly that you will be unable to work out and you'll be susceptible to sickness. Remember too that the weight you lose on such a regimen will only be partly fat and the rest muscle.

The only real way to lose the fat under your skin that hides muscular development is slowly and sensibly. Cut back on your total caloric intake by about 500 calories per day to lose one pound per week, and about 1000 calories per day to lose two pounds per week. Refer to some excellent books on nutrition and weight control listed in the appendix. As you work out, you will likely add some muscle tissue, so your weight may stay the same or actually increase, even though your body fat percentage decreases. The best way, then, to monitor fat loss is through the body fat determination procedure given earlier in this book, and not body weight per se.

Whatever nutritional play you design should stress variety and vegetables and whole-grain products. A varied diet will ensure that you get adequate amounts of all the nutrients your body needs. If you are one of those fortunate few who needs to gain weight, the slow, sensible approach will work best for you as well. Eat slightly higher amounts of complex carbohydrate foods and a bit more of the foods high in polyunsaturated fats (i.e., salad oil, margarine, etc.) and your weight gain will be largely muscle, assuming you are working out hard enough and eating sufficient protein to stimulate muscle growth. Make sure that you do not gain too much fat, though.

## SUPPLEMENTS—DO YOU NEED THEM?

If you are eating an adequate, varied diet that includes foods from the four basic food groups, it is unlikely that your body will be deficient in any vitamins or minerals. The need for vitamins has been highly exaggerated. Further, many vitamins, especially vitamin D and vitamin A, accumulate in the fatty tissues and can actually reach toxic levels in individuals who regularly consume high doses of vitamin supplements. If you feel that you need a supplement, choose one that has about 100 percent of all the essential B complex vitamins, which are not stored in large quantities in the body, and vitamins E and C.

Vitamins E and C may be special cases, because although the evidence is far from complete, small supplementary amounts of these vitamins may be physiologically useful. Vitamin C may or may not help reduce the severity of a cold, but it is essential for strong connective tissue growth and in the stabilization of many essential enzyme systems and other vitamins. Many physicians recommend that people take about 500 milligrams of vitamin C daily, as opposed to the recommended daily requirement of about 60 mg per day stated by the government. This added amount can come in foods, especially citrus juices, green vegetables, and, surprisingly, potatoes, or in tablet form. Megadoses of vitamin C should be avoided, though, because the body will adapt to this vitamin input and should you discontinue taking the supplement, your body can experience an artificial vitamin C deficiency.

Vitamin E is a factor necessary for the synthesis of some hormones and the stabilization of many biochemical reactions in the body, since it functions as an anti-oxidant. While the recommended daily requirement for vitamin E is 30 international units (IU), it may be wise to get about 100 IU per day. Such small supplementation seems to be healthful, although medical science really doesn't know why as yet. Again, megadoses of this vitamin are expensive and unwarranted. Remember, vitamins are simply catalysts for biochemical reactions and not magic bullets.

Although mineral deficiencies are usually not a problem for well-nourished individuals, you should be especially alert to include adequate calcium in your diet. Most adult women, in particular, do not get the recommended daily allowance (about 850 mg per day) of calcium, largely because they avoid dairy products in the erroneous belief that they are fattening. Four glasses of skim milk will supply this needed calcium, and low-fat dairy products are anything but fattening. Most Americans also consume large quantities of coffee and other fluids that promote calcium loss before it is absorbed in the intestines. Prolonged deficiency, however slight, in calcium in the diet results in calcium withdrawal from the bones. Many researchers currently believe that this negative calcium balance leads to the preponderance of brittle bone disease found in so many of our older citizens. Calcium also acts as a natural tranquilizer and its inclusion in the diet is vital for the gym athlete who is putting enormous stress on his nervous system. Make sure you get four or five servings of milk products or cheese daily—in low-fat form if you are watching calories. Certain bread products, canned fish, and tofu (soybean curd) are also high in calcium.

Nutrition, the vital basis for progress in the gym, should be approached just like your training, with dedication, but not fanaticism. Learn to be an informed consumer by reading product labels and nutritional literature, and you will have the essentials to sculpt your body into whatever you want it to be.

# Appendix I

## THE HEALTH CLUB CONTRACT: AN OVERVIEW

Here is a sample of the type of contract you will see if you decide to join a commercial health club. You need to be aware of the major points of this agreement in the same way you would if you were buying a new car. The contract you receive may differ slightly, but the main points will be the same.

Part A deals with the general rules and regulations governing the members' rights and obligations. Part B gives the specifics of the contract period itself. Especially important here is the termination and renewal date clause. Make certain that if you pay for a long-term membership, the dates are correct. "Card Number" in Part B refers to the membership card you will receive upon joining a club, Your membership card itself should also include information on the type of contract you signed, (i.e., long-term membership, one-year membership, etc.) and the expiration date of the contract. Part C is perhaps the most important section. It gives the terms of renewal. Further, each contract will have a clause similar to the "Notice" in Part C. It states that *you* are responsible for debt to a lending institution incurred through the financing of a health club contract. Under this disclosure clause, you may sue a health club that does not honor its part of the contract, to recover your money, but you are still liable for payments under a separate financial agreement. Some contracts will have a different "Notice Clause," which reads:

"Notice: any holder of this consumer credit contract is subject to all claims and defenses which the debtor could assert against the seller of memberships or services obtained pursuant hereto or with the proceeds hereof. Recovery hereunder by the debtor shall not exceed amounts paid by the debtor hereunder."

What this clause means is that you can notify the finance company and advise them you are refusing to make any further payments, should the club close, and pursuant to federal regulations, are invoking your right to preserve and assert all claims and defenses. Of course, if you do that, the finance company or bank may sue you for the debt and the courts will decide if you retain obligation for the debt in light of the club having closed. In any case, there is little to be gained by filing as a creditor against a bankrupt health club, but that may be your only legal recourse.

Part D deals with other rules and regulations that you will be obligated to under the contract and which the club agrees to render to you. Note especially clauses 8 and 10, which deal with illness or injury and its effect on the contract.

If you finance your membership, you will also have to fill out a finance agreement. This may be done right in the health club or through an outside agency. If you finance, make sure all details of financing, i.e., interest rates, monthly payments, total payments, etc., are fully indicated on the contract, just as you would for any major purchase. Be aware that you have three business days after signing a credit agreement or health club contract to cancel that agreement in full. Such notice must be sent by certified mail (see clause 10 of sample contract).

### Rules and Conditions for Use of Your Club
(including Rules and Conditions contained on the reverse side hereof)

1. HOURS OF OPERATION: The club's operating schedule may be changed from time to time. All clubs will be closed Sundays, holidays and from December 15 through and including January 1.

2. SIGNING IN: All Members upon entering club location are required to sign in at the sign-in counter, printing their name and membership card number. Member must present membership card and other suitable identification as requested by personnel in order to gain entrance into the club.

3. CHILDREN under twelve (12) years of age must be accompanied by an adult member at all times under supervision of club personnel.

4. GUEST PRIVILEGES: Members are invited to bring or send each of their friends to the Club for a complete treatment and figure or physique analysis as a free guest of the club, without cost or obligation to member or to guest. Member, subject to club manager's approval, can bring or send in as many guests as member so desires. However, the same friend may not come in as a guest more than one time in any twelve (12) month period. All guests must register at the desk and be under the complete supervision and guidance of an instructor.

5. EXERCISE CLOTHING: For Men: White gym shorts with T-shirt or sweat suit. White sweat sox or soft soled gym shoes must be worn at all times in the exercise area. For Women: Slacks, pedal pushers, slim jims, something of this nature that will not restrict freedom of movement in the exercises. Shorts are permissible, but not short shorts or loose fitting shorts. Flat shoes or white socks must be worn at all times in the exercise area.

6. TRANSFERS: No member of the Club shall advertise or permit their membership to be advertised for sale. Memberships are not transferable or assignable without written permission from the management.

---

Termination and
Contract Date _____ Renewal Date _____ Card No. _____

Mrs.
Mr.
Miss ————————————————————— Age ———————————

Spouse ——————————————————— Phone ———————————

Residence Address ————————————————————————————

City ————————————————— State ——————————— Zip ——————

Referred by: Member ——————————— Ad (type) ————— Other —————

---

RENEWAL: So long as the Member is in good standing Member may renew his membership each year for $ _____ per year paid in advance.

**NOTICE: If you are obtaining credit in connection with this purchase, you will be required to sign a promissory note, a sales contract or other instrument of indebtedness which may be purchased from the seller by a bank, finance company, or any other third party. If such is the case, you will be required to make your payments to someone other than the seller. You should be aware that if this happens you may have to pay the note, contract, or other instrument of indebtedness in full to its new owner even if your purchase contract is not fulfilled.**

I have read the "NOTICE" above and all of the Rules and Conditions contained on both sides of this paper. I accept and agree to be bound by these Rules and Conditions and acknowledge receiving a copy thereof.

_____
Buyer          (sign here)


_____
Buyer          (sign here)


By _____
    Signature of authorized person

### Additional Rules and Conditions of Membership

7. CONDUCT OF MEMBER: Members shall be subject to the control and guidance of the Club's staff while in the Club, and will follow instructions of the Club personnel. Members shall conduct themselves in a quiet, well-mannered fashion while in the club, and reserve all criticism of any major kind about Members, guests, Club, or Club personnel until in a private office with the Club Manager.

8. TERM OF MEMBERSHIP: Memberships shall be computed from the date of execution of the Member's contract and there shall be no abatement of the running of the specified term for any reason whatsoever, either by reason of a member's action or failure to act. In the event Member is unable to use the facilities because of illness or vacation, a maximum period of three months' "grace period" may be allowed at the option of the Club. This "grace period" will not apply to any payments. Failure to attend and use the club facilities does not relieve Member of any liability for payments and amounts due.

9. FACILITY USE: Except as prevented by act of God, war, strike, and other cause beyond its reasonable control, Club shall, during the term of Member's membership, maintain its facilities, the supervision thereof, and the hours during which they shall be available to Member substantially as of the date of this obligation. The Club may, however, at its option, supply and charge additionally for massage and towel rental. In the event that Member shall claim that his membership card is lost, stolen, or destroyed, the Club may require an affidavit setting forth the relevant circumstances and the payment of a $5.00 service fee before issuing a replacement card.

10. PHYSICAL HEALTH: Member may void this agreement within three (3) business days of the date of execution upon delivery by certified mail, return receipt requested, to seller, of a certificate from customer's (member's) physician that participation in seller's club program would impair the health of said customer during the term of said contract, provided such certificate is accurate and correct. Seller reserves the right to have an independent examination made of member to verify the accuracy and correctness of Member's physician's certificate.

11. USE OF FACILITIES BY MEMBERS: Member agrees and represents that exercises, treatments and use of all club facilities shall be undertaken at the Member's own risk, that he/she is in good physical condition and physically able to undertake any and all physical exercises and treatments provided by Club, and that the corporation which owns the Club and/or any affiliated companies and/or their respective agents and employees, shall not be liable for any claims, demands, injuries, damages, actions or causes of action, whatsoever, to Member or his or her property arising out of, or connected with the use of any of the services and/or facilities of such corporation and of any affiliated companies and/or their respective agents and employees, or the premises where the same are located, and the Member does hereby expressly forever release and discharge said corporation and any affiliated companies and their respective agents, and employees, from all such claims, demands, injuries, damages, actions, or causes or actions. In case of any accident, Member agrees and concedes that he will be examined at his sole expense by a licensed physician who shall report in writing to both member and the corporation owning the Club.

12. DAMAGE TO FACILITIES: Member agrees to pay an extra charge for damage arising from any careless use of equipment, or dropping of weights, etc. caused by Member. Should the Club or any facility therein be unavailable for Member's use due to damage by fire, act of God, catastrophe or accident or any other reason, at the sole option of Club, Member's membership time may be extended for a period equal to the time of such unavailability, or at the option of the Club, the member may be transferred to another Club within the same city. It is further agreed that the Club's entire premises may be closed or that Club's location may be changed, moved or eliminated in accordance with the expiration of leases or other management needs at the sole discretion of the Club, and Member agrees to accept the Club's decision as final. If a location is closed permanently, the Club will make every reasonable attempt to provide member with the rights to use another club within the geographical limits of the same city.

13. PERSONAL PROPERTY: The Club, the corporation owning the Club, and the agents and employees of the corporation owning the Club shall not be responsible for damaged, lost or stolen articles of clothing and other personal property of any member.

14. AMENDING OF RULES: The Club reserves the right to amend or add to these Rules and Conditions and to adopt new rules and conditions as it may deem necessary for the property management of the Club.

15. COMPLIANCE WITH RULES AND CONDITIONS: Member agrees to keep and obey all rules and conditions herein contained or in the future prescribed by the Club, and the Club reserves the right to revoke or terminate this membership if member fails to keep and obey any of such rules and conditions, and in this event, no part of Member's payments shall be refunded and any unpaid balance due from Member's membership in the Club, shall, at the election of the Club, become immediately due and payable.

16. WARRANTIES: Member agrees that no warranties, representations, or agreements of merchantibility, fitness for a particular purpose, or otherwise, express or implied, were made to member except for those written herein or in writing, signed by an officer of the corporation running the Club.

17. SEVERABILITY: If any provision of these Rules and Conditions is declared invalid or against public policy by a court of competent jurisdiction, the same shall be deemed not to have been included herein. All of the other provisions hereof shall continue in full force and effect and shall be interpreted to give, to the fullest extent possible, effect to the intent of the parties hereto as evidenced by the remaining provisions. If, any law or regulation requires the inclusion of provisions herein to validate this agreement, such provisions shall be deemed to be included, fully as if written herein. Anything herein to the contrary notwithstanding, if any provision herein is declared invalid or against public policy or if a provision not contained herein is required to be included to validate this agreement, and if the Club determines, in its sole discretion, that the exclusion or inclusion of such a provision imposes a burden upon the Club not contemplated by the Club when this membership was sold, the Club may, at its option, by giving written notice to the member cancel this membership agreement and be relieved of all obligation hereunder except to make the following payment to member: A sum of money which bears the same ratio

to 50% of the contract price of the entire membership as the unexpired portion of the membership period bears to the full term of this membership; provided that member has then paid all of his membership obligations. Said amount is so determined for the reason that the club incurs its greatest expenses on behalf of the member during the initial month of the membership.

18. DEFINITION: Whenever used herein, unless the context otherwise, requires, the word (a) "Member" shall mean the person signing as a "Buyer" or "Member" on the reverse side hereof, any purchaser of a club membership, any guest of a member using the Club, any person for whom a membership was purchased or made available, and all other persons using the Club and its facilities or services. All such persons, agree to be bound hereby as a condition precedent to their use of the club. (b) "Club" shall mean the corporation named at the bottom left hand side on the front of this document. (c) "Buyer" shall mean Member, except that where a person purchases a Membership for another, the purchasing person shall not be entitled to use club facilities and services, unless buyer has also purchased a Membership for Buyer.

# Appendix II

The following is a membership list of the International Physical Fitness Association, Inc. (I.P.F.A.) for the United States as of September 1981. IPFA was established in 1962 and is the world's largest health system, with 1500 affiliated fitness centers around the world. Membership in the IPFA entitles patrons of IPFA clubs certain privileges in transferring membership between IPFA affiliates and in other contractual matters.

IPFA international headquarters are at 415 W. Court St., Flint, Michigan 48503. Phone: (313) 239-2166.

## ALABAMA

**ANDALUSIA**
Solar Spa – Alt.
121 E. 3 Notch St.
Zip Code 36420
Ph. (205) 222-6561

**ANNISTON**
Cosmopolitan Spa, Int'l    Alt.
326 Blue Mountain Road, East
Zip Code 36201
Ph. (205) 237-4206

**AUBURN**
Kelly Lyn Figure Salon    Women
Corner Village Shopping Center
Dean Rd. and E. Glenn Ave.
Zip Code 36830
Ph. (205) 826-3600

**BIRMINGHAM**
International Figure    Women
7070 Weibel Drive (Fairfield)
Zip Code 35064
Ph. (205) 780-6200

International Figure, Inc.
Women
32 Green Springs Hwy.
Zip Code 35216
Ph. (205) 942-2250

International Figure, Inc.
Women
610 Lorna Rd./Lorna Square
P.O. Box 20252
Zip Code 35216
Ph. (205) 823-2702

International Figure, Inc.
Women
8512 Roebuck Pkwy. East
Zip Code 35206
Ph. (205) 833-3207

21st Century Health Spas    Dual
25th Avenue N.E.
Centerpoint Plaza
Zip Code 35215
Ph. (205) 859-4900

United Fitness Centers    Men
615 Lorna Square
Zip Code 35216
Ph. (205) 979-3067

**DECATUR**
Kelly Lyn Figure Salon    Women
Hills Plaza
2009 Beltline Rd. SW
Zip Code 35601
Ph. (205) 350-0772

World Olympic Health Spa, Inc.
2050 Beltline Hwy.
Zip Code 35601
Ph. (205) 350-1600

**DOTHAN**
Kelly Lyn Figure Salon    Women
Westgate Shopping Center
Zip Code 36303
Ph. (205) 793-1168

Renaissance Shape Spa    Alt.
Northside Mall
Zip Code 36301
Ph. (205) 794-6748

**ENTERPRISE**
Solar Spa of Enterprise    Alt.
4000 Fort Rucker Blvd.
Zip Code 36330
Ph. (205) 347-4353

**FOLEY**
Total Fitness Health Spa    Alt.
105 W. Berry Ave.
Zip Code 36535
Ph. (205) 943-4541

**HOOVER**
21st Century Health Spas    Dual
1580 Montgomery Hwy.
Zip Code 35216
Ph. (205) 979-6312

**HUNTSVILLE**
Kelly Lyn Figure Salon    Women
Parkway City Mall F7
2801 Memorial Parkway SW
Zip Code 35801
Ph. (205) 534-4514

21st Century Health Spa    Alt.
1963 Memorial Pkwy. Dunnavants
Zip Code 35801
Ph. (205) 539-8411

21st Century Health Spa    Alt.
Whitesburg Shopping Plaza
Zip Code 35802
Ph. (205) 881-2491

**IRONDALE**
21st Century Health Spas    Dual
Highway 78 East
Zip Code 35210
Ph. (205) 951-2192

**JACKSONVILLE**
Nautilus Health Club    Dual
26 Public Square
Zip Code 36265
Ph. (205) 435-6830

**LANGDALE**
Olympian Village Health Spa
Alt.
1807 44th St.
Zip Code 36864
Ph. (205) 756-2195

**MOBILE**
French Riviera Spa    Alt.
4363 Downtowner Loop North
Zip Code 36609
Ph. (205) 342-5093

Kelly Lyn Figure Salon    Women
254 Azalea Rd.
Zip Code 36609
Ph. (205) 344-0970

Shapely Lady Spa    Women
3963 Government Blvd.
Zip Code 36609
Ph. (205) 661-2622

**MONTGOMERY**
Figure Girl    Women
553 Northeastern Boulevard
Zip Code 36117
Ph. (205) 277-4471

Health Clubs of Montgomery
Dual
3824 Harrison Road    Perry Hill
Shop. Ctr.

Zip Code 36109
Ph. (205) 277-4978

Kelly Lyn Figure Salon    Women
311 B. McGeehee Rd.
Olde Town Shopping Center
Zip Code 36101
Ph. (205) 284-3305

Kelly Lyn Figure Salon    Women
East Montgomery Plaza
5439 Atlanta Hwy.
Zip Code 36117
Ph. (205) 279-1230

**OPELIKA**
Renaissance Fitness Centre    Alt.
107 N. 6th St.
Zip Code 36801
Ph. (205) 749-3362

**SARALAND**
The Ultimate Health Fitness &
Appearance, Inc.    Dual
211 Highway 43 South
Zip Code 36571
Ph. (205) 675-3336

**TUSCALOOSA**
Kelly Lyn Figure Salon    Women
2600 E. McFarland Blvd.
Zip Code 35401
Ph. (205) 345-8032

Nautilus Fitness Center    Dual
2135 University Blvd.
Zip Code 35401
Ph. (205) 758-8666

## ALASKA

**ANCHORAGE**
Nautilus of Alaska Fitness Center
Dual
307 E. Northern Lights Blvd.
Suite 201
Zip Code 99504
Ph. (907) 274-2718 or 277-7432

Spa Lady    Women
5437 E. Northern Lights Blvd.
Zip Code 99503
Ph. (907) 333-5556
Spa Lady    Women
500 W. Northern Lights Blvd.
Zip Code 99503
Ph. (907) 276-1863

## ARIZONA

**BISBEE**
Bisbee Health Studio – Alt.
81 Main Street, Box 1052
Zip Code 85603
Ph. (602) 432-2400

**GLENDALE**
Bell Tower Nautilus    Dual
6350 W. Bell Rd.
Zip Code 85308
Ph. (602) 979-0056

**MESA**
Fitness West – Dual
1440 W. Broadway
Zip Code 85202
Ph. (602) 898-0111

**PHOENIX**
Exclusively Women
1764 W. Bell Rd.
Zip Code 85023
Ph. (602) 993-1650

Exclusively Women
4015 No. 32nd St.
Zip Code 85018
Ph. (602) 957-9010

Exclusively Women Spas
5116 W. Northern Ave.
Zip Code 85302
Ph. (602) 931-3775

Gym & Swim   Alt.
3530 E. Thomas Road
Zip Code 85018
Ph. (602) 956-2200

Lovely Lady Exercise & Reducing
Salon   Women
3841 E. Thunderbird Rd.
Zip Code 85032
Ph. (602) 971-4166

Nautilus by the Pointe   Dual
7575 N. 16th St.
Zip Code 85020
Ph. (602) 944-5271

Nautilus 20 Minute Fitness Center
Dual
4041 N. Central Avenue, Suite
145
Zip Code 85012
Ph. (602) 241-9485

Paradise Valley Health Spa   Alt.
12428 N. Cave Creek Rd.
Zip Code 85022
Ph. (602) 971-3920

**SCOTTSDALE**
Nautilus Fitness Center   Dual
10320 N. Scottsdale Rd.
Zip Code 85253
Ph. (602) 991-4322

**SIERRA VISTA**
International Fitness Center   Alt
4341 S. Hwy 92
Zip Code 85635
Ph. (602) 378-2461

**TEMPE**
Grecian/Spa Fitness Center   Alt.
3400 S. Mill Ave.
Zip Code 85282
Ph. (602) 894-1263

**YUMA**
Yuma Racquet Club   Dual
3131 Winsor Ave.
Zip Code 85364
Ph. (602) 726-8386

## ARKANSAS

**FAYETTEVILLE**
Leon Snearly's Power Co.   Dual
427 N. College
Zip Code 72701
Ph. (501) 521-1153

Magic Mirror Figure Salon
Women
3332 N. College St.
Zip Code 72701
Ph. (501) 521-5100

Magic Mirror Roman Spa   Alt.
3322 N. College
Zip Code 72701
Ph. (501) 521-5100

**FORT SMITH**
Spa International Inc.   Alt.
180 Central Mall
Zip Code 72903
Ph. (501) 452-4410

**LITTLE ROCK**
French Riviera Spa   Alt.
University and "H" Streets
Zip Code 72205
Ph. (501) 555-0367

Fitness World   Women
11121 Rodney Parham
Zip Code 72211
Ph. (501) 224-9698

Kelly Lyn Figure Spa
Rodney Parham at I-430
Zip Code 72207
Ph. (501) 224-0935

Magic Mirror Figure Salon
Women
8211 Windameer
Zip Code 72209
Ph. 568-1378

National Health Spa   Alt.
3110 S. University
Zip Code 72204
Ph. (501) 568-3192

**NORTH LITTLE ROCK**
Fitness World   Women
3805 McCain Park
Zip Code 72116
Ph. (501) 753-3070

**PINE BLUFF**
Riverside Health Spa   Alt.
2407 Olive Street
Zip Code 71601
Ph. (501) 536-7260

**ROGERS**
The Body Shop   Dual
1810 S. 8th
Zip Code 72756
Ph. (501) 631-0424

World of Fitness   Women
1606 Southgate Shopping Center
Zip Code 72756
Ph. (501) 636-0376

**SPRINGDALE**
Leon Snearly's Power Company
Dual
1410 W. Sunset
Zip Code 72764
Ph. (501) 756-1153

## CALIFORNIA

**ANAHEIM**
Holiday Spa Health Club   Alt.
Playa Plaza Shopping Center
510 S. Beach Blvd.
Zip Code 92804
Ph. (714) 826-0381

**ANTIOCH**
Proud Woman Health Spa
Women
3658 Lone Tree Way

Zip Code 94509
Ph. (415) 754-9322

**ARCADIA**
Ultimate Fitness Center   Alt.
902 S. Bladwin
Zip Code 91006
Ph. (213) 445-6489

**BAKERSFIELD**
Jack LaLanne's Health Spa   Alt
1908 Nile St.
Zip Code 93305
Ph. (805) 497-9324

New World Health Club   Dual
809 Chester
Zip Code 93301
Ph. (805) 324-3736

**BONITA**
Spa Lady   Women
4348 Bonita Road
Zip Code 92002

**CAMERON PARK**
Cameron Park Health Club   Dual
3025 Alhambra Drive
Zip Code 95682
Ph. (916) 677-1681

**CAMPBELL**
Anastasias Fitness Center   Alt.
and Swim School
2931 S. Winchester Blvd.
Zip Code 95008
Py. (408) 379-8722

Walbangers Family Fitness &
Racquet Club   Alt.
577 Salmar Ave.
Zip Code 95008
Ph. (408) 379-6670

**CAPITOLA**

Capitola Spa Fitness Center –
Alt. & Co-ed
816 Bay Avenue
Zip Code 95010
Ph. (408) 475-6316

**CARLSBAD**
Exclusively Women Spa – Women
2626 El Camino Real
Zip Code 92008
Ph. (714) 729-7151

**CERRITOS**
Holiday Spa Health Club – Dual
11881 E. Del Amo Blvd.
Zip Code 90715
Ph. (213) 924-1514

**CHATSWORTH**
Holiday Spa Health Club – Dual
9143 DeSoto Ave.
Zip Code 91311
Ph. (213) 882-5912

**CHICO**
Jim Roberts Health Club – Alt.
260 E. First Street
Zip Code 95926
Ph. (916) 342-6931

**CHULA VISTA**
Family Fitness Centers – Dual
835 3rd Avenue
Zip Code 92010
Ph. (714) 425-6600

CLAIRMONT
Spa Lady – Women
Corner Genesse and Balbo
Genesse Shopping Center
Zip Code 91711
Ph. (714) 292-9669

CLAREMONT
Nautilus Fitness Center – Dual
P.O. Box 628
358 W. Foothill Blvd.
Zip Code 91711
Ph. (714) 621-9268

CONCORD
Win's Fitness World – Co-ed
1505 Willow Pass Rd.
Zip Code 94520
Py. (415) 827-1120

COSTA MESA
Bristol Nautilus Fitness Center –
Dual
3033 S. Bristol Ave.
Zip Code 82626
Ph. (714) 557-9861

Holiday Spa Health Club – Alt.
Harbor Shopping Center
2300 Harbor-Blvd.
Zip Code 92626
Ph. (714) 549-3368

Spa Lady – Women
2701 Harbor Blvd.
Zip Code 92626
Ph. (714) 540-9822

COVINA
The Ultimate Fitness Center
Dual
440 West Arrow Highway
Zip Code 91722
Ph. (213) 331-8208

CULVER CITY
The Fitness Factory – Women
6237 Bristol Parkway
Zip Code 90230
Ph. (213) 670-1380

Wallbangers Family Fitness &
Racquet Club – Alt.
19595 Pruneridge Ave.
Zip Code 95014
Ph. (408) 253-9090

CUPERTINO
First Lady Spa – Women
1265 Kentwood
Zip Code 95014
Ph. (408) 446-0898

DALY CITY
Wallbangers Family Fitness &
Racquet Club – Alt.
373 Gellert Blvd.
Zip Code 94015
Ph. (415) 994-1690

DOWNEY
Imperial Spa, Inc. – Dual
9440 E. Imperial Hwy.
Zip Code 90241
Ph. (213) 861-8241

DUBLIN
Dublin Health Spa – Dual
7151 Regional Street
Zip Code 94566
Ph. (415) 828-3713

EL CAJON
El Cajon Racquetball & Fitness
Center – Dual
526 Jamacha Road
Zip Code 92021
Ph. (714) 579-8004

Family Fitness Center – Dual
850 Anele Avenue
Zip Code 92020
Ph. (714) 442-0293

EL MONTE
Nautilus Plus – Dual
3380 Flair Dr., Suite 201
Zip Code 91731
Ph. (213) 280-2703

ENCINO
Holiday Spa Health Club – Dual
17031 Ventura Blvd.
Zip Code 91316
Ph. (213) 986-6330

ESCONDIDO
Exclusively Women Spa – Women
1320 E. Valley Pkwy.
Zip Code 92027
Ph. (714) 743-8000

FAIR OAKS
Joan Blake Austin – Dual
8510 Madison Ave.
Zip Code 95628
Ph. (916) 966-8444

FOSTER CITY
Wallbangers Family Fitness &
Racquet Club – Alt.
1159 Chess Dr.
Zip Code 94404
Ph. (415 573-6700

FOUNTAIN VALLEY
Imperial Spa, Inc. – Alt.
18030 Magnolia
Zip Code 92708
Ph. (714) 962-1388

Nautilus Plus of Fountain Valley
– Dual
8780 Warner Ave.
Zip Code 92708
Ph. (714) 847-3011

FRESNO
Cam II Fitness Center – Men
4207 N. Blackstone, Suite 212
Zip Code 93726
Ph. (209) 224-8323

Fair Lady Figure Salon – Women
4207 N. Blackstone, Suite 212
Zip Code 93726
Ph. (209) 224-8323

Universal Danae Health Spa – Alt.
6763 N. Cedar
Zip Code 93710
Ph. (209) 226-9680

FULLERTON
Crossroads Nautilus – Dual
3230 Yorba Linda Blvd.
Zip Code 92631
Ph. (714) 993-1100

GARDEN GROVE
Garden Square Health Club
Dual
9562 Garden Grove Blvd.
Zip Code 92644
Ph. (714) 537-5410

Imperial Spa Inc. – Dual
8251 Garden Grove Blvd.
Zip Code 92644
Ph. (714) 534-1472

Spa Lady – Women
9789 Chapman Ave.
Zip Code 92641
Ph. (714) 537-2800

HALF MOON BAY
Half Moon Bay Fitness Center
Dual
225 S. Cabrillo Hwy.
Top Floor, Bldg. D
Zip Code 94019
Ph. (415) 726-0530

HAYWARD
Continental Lady Spa
677 W. Tennyson Rd.
Zip Code 94544
Ph. (415) 782-8702

Golden Venus Health & Beauty
Spa – Women
21190 Hesperian Blvd.
Zip Code 94541
Ph. (415) 783-4500

Golden Venus Weight Room –
Dual
22540 Foothill Blvd.
Zip Code 94541
Ph. (415) 582-3380

Grecian Spas – Women
20812 Mission Blvd.
Zip Code 94544
Ph. (415) 276-0580

HOLLYWOOD
Holiday Spa Health Club – Dual
7080 Hollywood Blvd.
Zip Code 90028
Ph. (213) 469-6307

The Gym – Men
5919 Franklin Ave.
Zip Code 90028
Ph. (213) 462-9531

HUNTINGTON BEACH
Family Fitness Center – Dual
7454 Edinger St.
Zip Code 92047
Ph. (714) 847-7800

INGLEWOOD
Lovely Lady Figure Salon –
Women
11310 Crenshaw Blvd.
Zip Code 90303
Ph. (213) 754-2975

KENTFIELD
World Gym Marin — Dual
941 Sir Francis Drake Blvd.
Zip Code 94904
Ph. (415) 453-2300

LA HABRA
Imperial Spa, Inc. — Co-ed
1815 W. La Habra Blvd.
Zip Code 90631
Ph. (213) 694-1895

Nautilus Fitness Center — Alt.
323 N. Harbor Blvd.
Zip Code 90631
Ph. (213) 694-2034

LAKEWOOD
Family Fitness Center — Dual
4678 Daneland
Zip Code 90712
Ph. (213) 630-2668

LA MESA
Exclusively Women Spa — Women
8749 La Mesa Blvd.
Zip Code 92041
Ph. (714) 697-1222

Family Fitness Center — Dual,
Co-ed
7450 University Dr.
Zip Code 92041
Ph. (714) 697-1212

Spa Lady — Women
7590 El Cajon Blvd., Suite D
Zip Code 92041
Ph. (714) 461-0991

LIVERMORE
Grecian Spas — Co-ed
861 Rincon Ave.
Livermore Shopping Center
Zip Code 94550
Ph. (415) 443-3460

LONG BEACH
Holiday Spa Health Club — Alt.
4101 Atlantic Blvd.
Zip Code 90807
Ph. (213) 426-8874

LOS ALAMITOS
Aquarius Health Club — Alt.
10707 Bloomfield
Zip Code 90720
Ph. (213) 431-3503

LOS ANGELES
Nautilus Plus — Dual
818 W. 7th St.
Zip Code 90017
Ph. (213) 629-4336

Pacific Sports Clubs, Nautilus
Dual
8651 Lincoln Blvd.
Zip Code 90045
Ph. (213) 641-8023
     (213) 641-7796

World for Men Health Club
3283 Motor Ave.
Zip Code 90034
Ph. (213) 559-8350

LOS GATOS
First Lady Health Spa — Women
14107 Winchester Blvd.
Vasona Park Shopping Center
Zip Code 95031
Ph. (408) 866-7290

Tom Janis Health Club — Women
14120 Blossom Hill Rd.
Zip Code 95030
Ph. (408) 358-3377

MISSION VIEJO
Holiday Health Club Spa — Dual
22401 Alicia Parkway
Zip Code 92675
Ph. (714) 770-0822

MODESTO
Fitness Institute — Dual
2401 E. Orangeburg, Suite R
Zip Code 95355
Ph. (209) 524-6391

The Spa — Women
1700 McHenry Ave. No. 76F
Zip Code 95350
Ph. (209) 527-2561

MONTCLAIR
Holiday Spa Health Club — Alt.
5350 Olive St.
Zip Code 91763
Ph. (714) 626-3593

Spa Lady — Women
5007 S. Plaza Lane
Zip Code 91763
Ph. (714) 621-6769

MONTEREY
Club Monterey — Dual
656 Munras Ave.
Zip Code 93940
Ph. (408) 646-9648

Del Monte Spa Fitness Center —
Alt.
290 Del Monte Center
Zip Code 93940
Ph. (408) 373-3793

Emperor & Empress Health Spa —
Alt.
1100 So. Atlantic
Zip Code 91754
Ph. (213) 570-9723

MORAGA
The Proud Woman Health Spa —
Women
370 Park Street
Zip Code 94556
Ph. (415) 375-6535

MOUNTAIN VIEW
First Lady Spa — Women
830 El Camino Real
Zip Code 94040
Ph. (408) 738-2086

Wallbangers Family Fitness &
Racquet Club — Alt.
2535 Showers Dr.
Zip Code 94040
Ph. (415) 948-4400

NAPA
Napa Health Studio — Dual
2414 Jefferson St.
Zip Code 94558
Ph. (707) 255-6767

Proud Women Health Spa —
Women
638 Trancas St.
Zip Code 94558
Ph. (707) 226-1874

NEWPORT BEACH
Lido Nautilus — Dual
3295 Newport Blvd.
Zip Code 92663
Ph. (714) 675-1171

NORTHRIDGE
Nautilus Plus — Dual
8948 Corbin
Zip Code 91324
Ph. (213) 885-7417

OAKLAND
Golden Venus Health & Beauty
Spa — Women
5136 Broadway
Zip Code 94611
Ph. (415) 652-9232

Golden Venus Health & Figure
Spa — Women
10700 MacArthur Blvd.
Zip Code 94605
Ph. (415) 562-8554

OCEANSIDE
Family Fitness Centers — Dual
2213 E. Camino Real
Zip Code 92054
Ph. (714) 439-4404

ORANGE
Holiday Spa Health Club — Alt.
Plaza Real Shopping Center
622 E. Katella Ave.
Zip Code 92667
Ph. (714) 639-2441

PALMS
World for Women Health Club &
Spa — Women
34404 Motor Avenue
Zip Code 90034
Ph. (213) 839-4311

PLEASANT HILL
Continental Lady Spa — Women
220 Golf Club Rd.
Zip Code 94523
Ph. (415) 676-0858

Golden Venus Health & Beauty
Spa — Women
No. 1 Mayhew Way
Zip Code 94523
Ph. (415) 932-4844

Lovely Lady Health Spa —
Women
2625 Pleasant Hill Rd.
Zip Code 94523
Ph. (415) 935-4895

POMONA
    International Health Spa — Alt.
    2449 N. Garey Ave.
    Zip Code 91767
    Ph. (714) 593-2583

    Pacific Coast Gym — Alt.
    1065 E. Holt Ave.
    Zip Code 91766
    Ph. (714) 622-9271

    Western Racquetball and Fitness
    Center — Dual
    275 E. Foothill Blvd.
    Zip Code 91767
    Ph. (714) 596-1834

POWAY
    Exercise Unlimited Inc. — Dual
    12635 Poway Rd.
    Zip Code 90264
    Ph. (714) 486-2544

RANCHO CORDOVA
    Cordova Gym/Patricia Ann Figure
    Salon — Dual
    10357 Folsom Blvd.
    Zip Code 95670
    Ph. (916) 363-6584

    Continental Lady Spa — Women
    2826 Zinfandel Dr.
    Zip Code 95670
    Ph. (916) 635-8530

REDWOOD CITY
    Dennis Nelson's Health Spa —
    Dual
    515 Veterane Blvd.
    Zip Code 94063
    Ph. (415) 365-3800

RESEDA
    Valley Gym & Health Club — Alt.
    7110 Reseda Blvd.
    Zip Code 91335
    Ph. (213) 705-9074

RIVERSIDE
    Holiday Spa Health Club — Alt.
    4020 Madison
    Zip Code 92504
    Ph. (714) 687-1315

    Joni's California Health Spa —
    Alt.
    3644 University Ave.
    Zip Code 92501
    Ph. (714) 683-3871

    Spa Lady — Women
    10120 Magnolia Ave.
    Zip Code 92503
    Ph. (714) 785-5220

ROLLING HILL ESTATES
    Palos Verdes Health Spas — Alt.
    720 Deep Valley Dr.
    Zip Code 90274
    Ph. (213) 377-9044

ROSEVILLE
    Joan Blake Austin — Dual
    1016 Douglas Blvd.
    Zip Code 95678
    Ph. (916) 782-7726

SACRAMENTO
    Fitness Institute — Dual
    2535 Fair Oaks Blvd.
    Zip Code 95825
    Ph. (916) 483-6011

SALINAS
    Northridge Spa Fitness Center —
    Alt. & Co-ed
    578 Northridge Shopping Center
    Zip Code 93906
    Ph. (408) 443-1021

SAN BERNARDINO
    Arrowhead Athletic Club — Dual
    1275 E. Highland Ave.
    Zip Code 92404
    Ph. (714) 886-6803

    The Body Factory - Dual
    25384 Baseline
    Zip Code 92410
    Ph. (714) 884-3598

    Holiday Spa Health Club — Dual
    333 North "H" Street
    Zip Code 92410
    Ph. (714) 888-1361

    Nautilus of San Bernardino
    Dual
    480 W. Court St.
    Zip Code 92401
    Ph. (714) 884-7251

SAN DIEGO
    Bill Pearl's Fitness Center — Dual
    7190 Miramar Rd., Suite 5
    Zip Code 92126
    Ph. (714) 578-1360

    Exclusively Women Spas
    670 University
    Zip Code 92107
    Ph. (714) 294-9111

    Family Fitness Center — Dual
    4405 La Jolla Village Dr.
    Zip Code 92122
    Ph. (714) 457-3930

    Family Fitness Centers — Dual
    5885 Rancho Mission Rd.
    Zip Code 92108
    Ph. (714) 281-5543

    Family Fitness Center — Dual
    7620 Balboa Ave.
    Zip Code 92111
    Ph. (714) 292-5539

    Family Fitness Center — Dual
    3345 Midway Drive
    Zip Code 92110
    Ph. (714) 224-2902

SAN FRANCISCO
    Golden Venus Health & Beauty
    Spa — Women
    2001 Van Ness Ave.
    Zip Code 94109
    Ph. (415) 885-4556

SAN GABRIEL
    Ultimate Fitness Center — Women
    606 W. Las Tunas Blvd.
    Zip Code 91775
    Ph. (213) 576-9262

    Ultimate Fitness Center — Men
    114 W. Valley Blvd.
    Zip Code 91776
    Ph. (213) 280-9160

SAN JOSE
    Grecian Spas — Co-ed
    1818 Hillsdale Ave.
    Zip Code 95124
    Ph. (408) 265-2081

    Grecian Spas — Co-ed
    5299 Prospect Road
    Zip Code 95129
    Ph. (408) 255-6585

SAN MATEO
    Continental Lady Spa — Women
    302 E. 4th Avenue
    Zip Code 94401
    Ph. (415) 344-1157

    San Mateo Fitness Center — Dual
    1743 S. El Camino Real
    Zip Code 94402
    Ph. (415) 574-4999

SAN PEDRO
    Palos Verdes Health Spa of San
    Pedro — Alt.
    28046 Western Avenue
    Zip Code 90732
    Ph. (213) 548-6226

SANTA ANA
    Spa Lady — Women
    2231 N. Tustin
    Zip Code 92701
    Ph. (714) 547-4453

SANTA BARBARA
    Pepitone Health Spa — Women
    3889 LaCumbre Plaza Lane
    Zip Code 93105
    Ph. (805) 687-0781

SANTA CRUZ
    Santa Cruz Health Club — Dual
    1212 17th Ave.
    Zip Code 95062
    Ph. (408) 462-2544

SANTEE
    Exclusively Women Spa — Women
    9720 Cyamaca
    Zip Code 92071
    Ph. (714) 449-2002

    Lance Alworth Family Fitness
    Center — Dual
    9635 15 Mission Gorge Rd.
    Zip Code 92071
    Ph. (714) 562-1666

SHERMAN OAKS
    Coldwater Chandler Racquetball
    Center — Dual
    5300 Coldwater Canyon Ave.
    Zip Code 91491
    Ph. (213) 985-8686

    World for Women — Women
    15451 Ventura Blvd.
    Zip Code 91403
    Ph. (213) 986-6991

SIMI VALLEY
    Ann Wynn's Spa Health Club (The
    Spa ) — Women
    2264 Tapo Street
    Zip Code 93063
    Ph. (805) 522-3248

SOQUEL
Santa Cruz Spa Fitness Center
Alt. & Co-ed
2710 – 41st Ave.
Zip Code 95073
Ph. (408) 476-7373

STOCKTON
Crystal Springs Health World –
Dual
1212 E. Hammer Lane
Zip Code 95210
Ph. (209) 957-9653

Grecian Spas – Co-ed
960 W. Robinhood Dr.
Zip Code 95207
Ph. (209) 477-4434

SUISUN
Mens Life/Ladies Life Health Spa
–Dual
311 Spring St.
Zip Code 94585
Ph. (707) 422-9776

SUNNYVALE
Sunnyvale Fitness Center – Dual
425 Indio Avenue
Zip Code 94086
Ph. (408) 746-0488

THOUSAND OAKS
Jack LaLanne Health Spa    Alt.
593 Moorpart Rd.
Zip Code 91360
Ph. (805) 324-9718

TORRANCE
Holiday Spa Health Club    Dual
20040 Hawthorne Blvd.
Zip Code 90503
Ph. (213) 542-3511

VAN NUYS
Coast & Valley Health Spas
Alt.
8638 Woodman Ave.
Zip Code 91331
Ph. (213) 893-8466

VENTURA
Coast & Valley Health Spa
3530 E. Main St.
Zip Code 93003
Ph. (805) 642-0197

WALNUT CREEK
Win's Fitness World – Alt.
1817 Ygnacio Valley Road
Zip Code 94598
Ph. (415) 938-4252

WEST LOS ANGELES
Holiday Spa Health Club – Dual
1914 South Bundy Dr.
Zip Code 90025
Ph. (213) 820-7571

WESTMINISTER
Holiday Spa Health Club – Dual
Westminister Center
6757 Westminister Ave.
Zip Code 92683
Ph. (714) 894-3387

WHITTIER
Imperial Spa Inc.    Alt.
15334 E. Whittier Blvd.
Zip Code 90603
Ph. (213) 948-6728

Nautilus National Health Club –
Co-ed
14320 E. Telegraph
Zip Code 90604
Py. (213) 941-3289

WOODLAND HILLS
World for Women Health Club &
Spa – Women
19739 Ventura Blvd.
Zip Code 91634
Ph. (213) 999-5415

YUBA CITY
Fitness Institute    Alt.
704 Onstott
Zip Code 95991
Ph. (916) 674-7400

LITTLETON
Nautilus Fitness Center    Dual
5120 S. Lowell
Zip Code 80014
Ph. (303) 794-7237

Patricia J's Women's Spa
Women
5151 S. Federal Blvd.
Zip Code 80123
Ph. (303) 795-8800

NORTHGLENN
Figurama – Women
826 E. 104th Ave.
Zip Code 80233
Ph. (303) 457-4051

Spa Lady – Women
960 W. 104th Ave.
Zip Code 80236
Ph. (303) 451-8696

PUEBLO
Pueblo Physical Fitness Center –
Dual
4025 Fortino Blvd.
Northgate Plaza Shopping Center
Zip Code 81008
Ph. (303) 543-1716

WHEATRIDGE
American Gym    Dual
4515 Harlan
Zip Code 80033
Ph. (303) 421-9660

## CONNECTICUT

AVON
American Health Fitness Centers
Alt.
353 West Main St.
Zip Code 06001
Ph. (203) 677-5277

BRANFORD
American Health Fitness Center
Alt.
Branhaven Plaza, Rt. 1
1060 W. Main Street
Zip Code 06405
Ph. (203) 481-4293

CROMWELL
Courtside At Cromwell    Dual
10 Hillside Rd.
Zip Code 06416
Ph. (203) 635-5400

ENFIELD
American Health Fitness Center
Alt.
85 Freshwater Blvd.
Zip Code 06082
Ph. (203) 623-6173

GLASTONBURY
The Active Woman Health & Fit-
ness Center – Dual
2840 Main Street
Zip Code 06033
Ph. (203) 633-3615

HAMDEN
American Health Fitness Centers
–Alt.
3025 Fixwell Ave.
Zip Code 06518
Ph. (203) 248-9391

HARTFORD
American Health Fitness Center
–Dual
Prospect Plaza
32-34 Kane St.
West Hartford
Zip Code 06119
Ph. (203) 233-1238

American Health Fitness Center
–Dual
60 Washington St., Suite 300
Zip Code 06106
Ph. (203) 246-7276

MANCHESTER
American Health Fitness Centers
515 Middleturnpike Section
Zip Code 06040
Ph. (203) 646-4260

American Lady Fitness Center of
Manchester, Inc. – Women
434 Oakland St.
Zip Code 06040
Ph. (203) 649-1611

MILFORD
American Health Fitness Centers
–Alt.
233 Broad St. North
Zip Code 06460
Ph. (203) 877-0367

NORWALK
Executive Spa, Inc. –Alt.
416 Westport Ave.
Zip Code 06851
Ph. (203) 846-3221

SOUTHINGTON
American Lady Fitness Center of
Southington, Inc. – Women
Caldor Village, Queen St.
Zip Code 06489

TORRINGTON
Woman's World Health Spas –
Women
Torrington Parkade
Winsted Road
Zip Code 06790
Ph. (203) 482-0277 or 489-0273

WATERBURY
American Health Fitness Centers
– Alt.
1525 Hamilton Ave.
Zip Code 06706
Ph. (203) 757-9267

WETHERSFIELD
American Health Fitness Center
Alt.
1199 Silas Deane Hwy.
Zip Code 06109
Ph. (203) 563-8167

## DELAWARE

CLAYMONT
Kirkwood Fitness Club    Alt.
99 Naamans Rd.
Zip Code 19703
Ph. (302) 798-1441

GREENVILLE
Greenville Racquetball Club
Dual
3704 Kennett Pike
Zip Code 19808
Ph. (302) 654-2473

NEWARK
Kirkwood Fitness Club    Dual
1750 Capitol Trail
Zip Code 19711
Ph. (302) 737-6877

## FLORIDA

ALTAMONTE SPRINGS
Mademoiselle    Women
515 E. Altamonte Dr.
Zip Code 32701
Ph. (305) 331-7602

Nautilus Fitness of Seminole –
Alt.
499 W. Hwy 434
San Sebastian Square
Zip Code 32701
Ph. (305) 862-1191

BOCA RATON
Future Shapes    Women
1287 W. Palmetto Park Rd.
Zip Code 33432
Ph. (305) 395-7991

CAPE CORAL
Jack LaLanne's Total Fitness
Center Inc.    Dual
850 Lafayette St.
Zip Code 33904
Ph. (813) 939-3858

CASSELBERRY
Holiday Health Spa & Fitness
Club    Alt.
1441 E. Semoran Boulevard
Zip Code 32707
Ph. (305) 678-0007

CLEARWATER
Lemon Tree International Health
Spa – Dual
920 So. Myrtle Avenue
Zip Code 33516
Ph. (813) 441-8411

Louisa International    Women
1665 Gulf to Bay Blvd.
Zip Code 33516
Ph. (813) 447-4591

Monarch Health Spas    Women
1163 N. Hercules Ave.
Zip Code 33515
Ph. (813) 442-0404

CORAL GABLES
My Fair Lady Salon    Women
275 University Dr.
Zip Code 33134
Ph. (305) 443-7467

Vic Tanny of Florida, Inc.    Alt.
1120 Ponce de Leon
Zip Code 33134
Ph. (305) 445-7764

CRESTVIEW
Solar Spa of Crestview – Alt.
1001 S. Ferdon Blvd.
Zip Code 32536
Ph. (904) 682-5106

DADELAND
Vic Tanny of Florida    Alt.
9215 S. Dixie Hwy.
Zip Code 32720
Ph. (305) 661-4256

DAVIE
Nautilus Nutrition & Fitness
Center, Inc.    Dual
4627 University Dr.
Davie Shopping Center
Zip Code 33328
Ph. (305) 434-7200

DAYTONA BEACH
National Health Studios    Alt.
1312 Volusia Ave.
Zip Code 32014
Ph. (904) 252-5557

DELRAY BEACH
Delray Nautilus Fitness Center
Alt.
1672 S. Federal Hwy.
Zip Code 33444
Ph. (305) 278-7111

FORT LAUDERDALE
American Spa Fitness Centers
Dual
1001 W. Oakland Park Blvd.
Zip Code 3331
Ph. (305) 561-3804

My Fair Lady    Women
4850 W. Oakland Park Blvd.
Zip Code 33313
Ph. (305) 485-7474

Vic Tanny of Florida, Inc.    Alt.
3801 N. Federal Hwy.
Zip code 31906
Ph. (305) 565-4658

Vic Tanny-European
5990 N. Federal Hwy.
Zip Code 33308
Ph. (305) 491-5400

FORT MYERS
Global Health Spa    Alt.
1916 Commercial Drive
Zip Code 33901
Ph. (813) 936-7356

Total Fitness Center, Inc. – Dual
4224 Fowler St.
Zip Code 33901
Ph. (813) 939-3858

FORT WALTON BEACH
Casey's Fitness Center – Men
25 Racetrack Rd.
Zip Code 32548
Ph. (904) 863-2800

Nationwide Fitness Spa – Alt.
4 Racetrack Rd., N.W.
Zip Code 32548
Ph. (904) 242-3110

Rene's Figure Spa    Women
128 Racetrack Road
Zip Code 32548
Ph. (904) 585-8085

HIALEAH
My Fair Lady    Women
4680 W. 17th Court
Zip Code 33020
Ph. (305) 822-7171

Vic Tanny of Florida, Inc.    Alt.
975 W. 49th Street
Zip Code 33012

HOLLYWOOD
Hollywood Spa & Health Club
Inc.    Alt.
6712 Stirling Rd.
Zip Code 33024
Ph. (305) 981-9633

Vic Tanny of Florida, Inc.    Alt.
2736 Hollywood Blvd.
Zip Code 33020
Ph. (305) 923-8417

HOMESTEAD
Vita-Lady health Spa    Women
887 NE 8th St.
Zip Code 33030
Ph. (305) 245-8845

INDIATLANTIC
Teri's 5th Ave. Spa    Alt.
203 5th Ave.
Zip Code 32903
Ph. (305) 725-3438

JACKSONVILLE
American Fitness Center – Dual
7500 Beach Blvd.
Zip Code 32216
Ph. (904) 721-2105

National Health Spa – Alt.
5515 Norwood Ave.
Zip Code 32208
Ph. (904) 764-5595

National Health Spa – Alt.
4467 Roosevelt Blvd.
Zip Code 32210
Ph. (904) 387-5608

National Health Spa – Dual
6494 Ft. Caroline Rd.
Zip Code 32211
Ph. (904) 743-6111

National Health Spa    Alt.
2050 S. Third St.
Zip Code 32250
Ph. (904) 246-9918

KENDALL
  Fitness Factory    Dual
  8100 SW 81st Dr.
  Kings Creek Village Shopping
  Plaza
  Zip Code 33143
  Ph. (305) 595-1234

LAKE CITY
  Uni Spa II    Men & Women
  1751 Hwy. 90 W.
  Zip Code 32055

LAKELAND
  Holiday Spa Lady    Alt.
  Lakeland Mall No. 58
  Zip Code 33801
  Ph. (813) 688-8785

LAKE WORTH
  Future Shapes of Lake Worth
  Women
  2525 N. Dixie Hwy.
  Zip Code 33460
  Ph. (305) 585-8085

LAUDERDALE-BY THE-SEA
  Nautilus-By-The-Sea    Dual
  4345 E. Tradewinds Ave.
  Zip Code 33308
  Ph. (305) 491-4969

LAUDERHILL
  Vic Tanny International    Alt.
  1172 N.W. 40th Ave.
  Zip Code 33313
  Ph. (305) 792-2525

LEESBURG
  Leesburg Health Studio    Alt.
  101 East Main St.
  Zip Code 32748
  Ph. (904) 787-2418

LIGHTHOUSE POINT
  Nautilus Fitness Club    Dual
  5000 N. Federal Hwy.
  Zip Code 33064
  Ph. (305) 428-5200

LONGWOOD
  The Fitness Force Nautilus
  Alt.
  190 Wekiva Springs Rd.
  Zip Code 32750
  Ph. (305) 862-1191

MAITLAND
  Holiday Health Spa & Fitness
  Club    Alt.
  1780 Park Avenue North
  Zip Code 32751
  Ph. (305) 644-2444

  Holiday Spa & Fitness Club
  Women
  501 George Ave.
  Zip Code 32751
  Ph. (305) 647-6400

MERRITT ISLAND
  Teri's Fitness Center    Alt.
  670 N. Courtenay Pky.
  Zip Code 32952
  Ph. (305) 452-5673

MIAMI
  My Fair Lady    Women
  12N 2 Biscayne Blvd.
  Zip Code 33132
  Ph. (305) 893-0216

My Fair Lady    Women
19181 S. Dixie Hwy.
Zip Code 33157
Ph. (305) 255-4400

My Fair Lady    Women
9655 S. Dixie Hwy.
Zip Code 33156
Ph. (305) 666-6187

Universal Health Studio    Dual
5345 S.W. 8th Street
Zip Code 33134
Ph. (305) 443-1632

Vic Tanny of Florida    Alt.
9205 S. Dixie Highway
Dadeland Area
Zip Code 33156

NAPLES
  Executive Health Spa    Alt.
  Naples Shopping Center
  2073 9th St. North
  Zip Code 33940
  Ph. (813) 261-1188

NICEVILLE
  Solar Spa    Alt.
  1031 Palm Plaza
  Zip Code 32578
  Ph. (904) 678-1141

NORTH MIAMI
  Vic Tanny of Florida, Inc.    Alt.
  1190 N.E. 163rd St.
  1190 Building
  Zip Code 33169
  Ph. (305) 949-6146

NORTH PALM BEACH
  Universal Spas of N. Palm Beach,
  Inc.    Alt.
  124 U.S. Highway One
  Zip Code 33408
  Ph. (305) 842-2404

ORANGE PARK
  National Health Spa    Alt.
  554 Kingsley Ave.
  Zip Code 32073
  Ph. (904) 264-7523

ORLANDO
  Holiday Health Spa & Fitness
  Club    Alt.
  3326 Edgewater Dr.
  Edgewater
  Zip Code 32032
  Ph. (305) 422-8176

  Holiday Health Spa & Fitness
  Club – Alt.
  450 E. Compton
  Zip Code 32806
  Ph. (305) 425-0538

  Nautilus Fitness Center of S.
  Orlando – Co-ed
  6220 S. Orange Blossom Tr.
  (Suite 605)
  Zip Code 32809
  Ph. (305) 857-2271

ORMOND BEACH
  National Health Spa – Alt.
  Trails Shopping Center
  Zip Code 32074
  Ph. (904) 672-7246

PANAMA CITY
  Springfield Spa & Racquetball
  Club – Alt. . . . . . . . . . . . . . .
  P.O. Box 3508
  3203 E. Business Hwy. 98
  Zip Code 32401
  Ph. (904) 769-3545

PENSACOLA
  Body College & Fitness Center
  Alt.
  710 N. Alcantz St.
  Zip Code 32501
  Ph. (904) 434-3035

  Isadora Spa    Women
  Cordova Mall
  Zip Code 32504
  Ph. (904) 477-9476

  Renaissance Fitness Spa    Dual
  4477 Mobile Hwy.
  Zip Code 32506
  Ph. (904) 455-3902

PLANTATION
  Bodyworks    Dual
  1755 N. University Dr.
  Zip Code 33324
  Ph. (305) 472-4399

  My Fair Lady    Women
  7077 W. Broward Blvd.
  Zip Code 33317
  Ph. (305) 791-9600

  Vic Tanny-European
  601 N. State Road, No. 7
  Zip Code 33317
  Ph. (305) 791-4710

POMPANO
  Vic Tanny of Florida, Inc.    Alt.
  1650 N. Federal Hwy.
  Zip Code 33062
  Ph. (305) 781-7440

ST. PETERSBURG
  Lemon Tree International Health
  Spa    Dual
  4600 4th Street North
  Zip Code 33703
  Ph. (813) 522-5505

  Louisa International – Women
  5651 38th Ave., North
  Zip Code 33710
  Ph. (813) 381-7841

  Sunshine Health & Fitness Center
  Alt.
  7995 8th St., North
  Zip Code 33702
  Ph. (813) 577-2004

SOUTH MIAMI
  Bodyworks    Dual
  5950 Sunset Dr.
  Zip Code 33143
  Ph. (305) 665-5468

SOUTH PASADENA
  Lemon Tree International Health
  Spa    Alt.
  6882 Gulfport Blvd. South
  Pasadena Shopping Center
  Zip Code 33707
  Ph. (813) 384-0575

STUART
Universal Spas of Stuart, Inc.
Alt.
2461 E. Ocean Blvd.
Zip Code 33494
Ph. (305) 283-6066

TALLAHASSEE
The Spa (TransAmerican Health
Spa) — Alt.
2415 N. Monroe Ut. 290. Talla-
hassee Mall
Zip Code 32303

TAMPA
Boddy Shoppe Gym — Dual
3922 W. Hillsborough Ave.
Zip Code 33614
Ph. (813) 877-9757

Carrollwood Fitness — Dual
12420 N. Dale Mabry
Zip Code 33618
Ph. (813) 962-2718

Lady Athena Spa — Women
3706 W. Waters Ave.
Zip Code 33614
Ph. (815) 933-4979

Louisa International — Women
9390 N. Florida Ave.
Zip Code 33612
Ph. (813) 933-2864

Louisa International — Women
3808 Swann Ave.
Zip Code 33609
Ph. (813) 872-8427

Sum Figure of Tampa — Women
6702 Hanley Rd.
Zip Code 33614
Ph. (813) 886-2560

TEQUESTA
Universal Spas of Tequesta, Inc.
Alt.
383 Tequesta Dr.
Zip Code 33458
Ph. (305) 746-9268

WEST PALM BEACH
Future Shapes of West Palm
Beach — Women
4645 Gun Club Road
Zip Code 33406
Ph. (305) 689-9568

Universal Spas of W. Palm Beach,
Inc. — Alt.
7627 S. Dixie Highway
Zip Code 33406
Ph. (305) 585-9305

Vic Tanny-European
1615 Palm Beach Lake Blvd.
Zip Code 33401
Ph. (305) 686-5055

## GEORGIA

ALBANY
Nautilus Fitness Center — Dual
1113 Whispering Pine Rd.
Zip Code 31701
Ph. (912) 883-5290

ATHENS
Spa South of Georgia — Alt.
820 Hawthorne Ave.
Zip Code 30604
Ph. (404) 549-2517

ATLANTA
American Fitness Center — Alt.
6780 Roswell Rd., NW
Zip Code 30328
Ph. (404) 394-0090

Fitness 1st N.E. — Co-ed
1407 Peachtree Street, N.E.
Zip Code 30309
Ph. (404) 881-1718

My Fair Lady Salon — Women
5944 Roswell Road, NE
Zip Code 30328
Ph. (404) 255-8560

My Fair Lady Salon — Women
3549-C Chamblee Tucker
Zip Code 30341
Ph. (404) 455-8385

Olympic World Gym — Dual
6315 Roswell Rd.
Zip Code 30328
Ph. (404) 252-3219

Norwegian Health Spa — Alt.
3210 Northlake Pkwy.
Zip Code 30345
Ph. (404) 934-1010

AUGUSTA
The Augusta Spa & Racquet Club
Alt.
Southgate Plaza, Ft. Gordon Hwy.
Zip Code 30906
Ph. (404) 736-2566

Nautilus of Augusta Health Center
— Dual
2825 Washington Rd., Fairway
Square
Zip Code 30909
Ph. (404) 738-2529

Spa Lady Fitness Center —
Women
1758 Gordon Rd.
Zip Code 30904
Ph. (404) 738-8913

Spa Lady Fitness Center —
Women
2825 Washington Rd.
Zip Code 30907
Ph. (404) 738-8716

Spa Fitness Center — Men
3122 Wrightsboro Rd.
Zip Code 30909
Ph. (404) 738-0635

BRUNSWICK
Nautilus Fitness Center — Dual
4999 Altama Avenue
Zip Code 31520
Ph. (912) 264-6958

CALHOUN
Southern Fitness Centers of
America, Inc. — Alt.
434 South Wall St.
Zip Code 30701
Ph. (404) 629-9101

CARTERSVILLE
Cartersville Health Spa — Alt.
228 S. Tennessee St.
Zip Code 30120
Ph. (404) 382-7443

COLLEGE PARK
Fitness Center — Nautilus Karate
— Alt.
6159 Old National Hwy.
Zip Code 30349
Ph. (404) 997-7496

COLUMBUS
Nautilus Fitness Center — Dual
2505 Airport Thruway
Simons Plaza
Zip Code 31904
Ph. (404) 322-0260

Olympic Health Spa — Men
2435 Wynnton Road
Zip Code 31906
Ph. (404) 327-9381

Olympic Health Spa — Women
1216 Stark Ave.
Zip Code 31906
Ph. (404) 322-9322

CONYERS
Nautilus Health Club — Alt.
2180 Salem Rd.
Fieldstone Mall
Zip Code 30208
Ph. (404) 922-5470

DALTON
Europa Health Spa — Alt.
Cleveland Hwy. — Whitfield
Square
Zip Code 30720
Ph. (404) 278-7734

Health World International — Alt.
Dalton Shopping Center
West Walnut Avenue
Zip Code 30720
Ph. (404) 278-0773

Kelly Lyn Figure Salons —
Women
111K Bryman Plaza, N.
Zip Code 30720
Ph. (404) 278-8031

DECATUR
My Fair Lady Beauty Retreat &
Figure Salon — Women
82 S. DeKalb Mall
Zip Code 30034
Ph. (404) 243-1055

DORAVILLE
Fitness for Life America — Dual
5803 Buford Hwy.
Zip Code 30340
Ph. (404) 458-1800

DOUGLASVILLE
Eternal Youth Health Spa — Alt.
8218 Dura Lee Lane
Zip Code 30134
Ph. (404) 949-3721

ELLIJAY
World of Fitness — Alt.
14 Gilmer Shopping Center
Zip Code 30540
Ph. (404) 635-7451

**FOREST PARK**
Spa Lady Fitness Center –
Women
Forest Park Shopping Center
442 Jonesboro Rd.
Zip Code 30050
Ph. (404) 363-2753

**FORT OGLETHORPE**
John Allen's Roman Spa – Alt.
Highway 2A
Zip Code 30742
Ph. (404) 866-9570

**GAINESVILLE**
Lanier Spa, Inc.  Alt.
Lakeshore Mall
Zip Code 30501
Ph. (404) 536-3232

**JONESBORO**
American Fitness Center   Alt.
6439 Tara Blvd.
Zip Code 30236
Ph. (404) 477-8820

U.S.A. Fitness World   Alt.
8643 Tara Blvd.
Zip Code 30236
Ph. (404) 471-8360

**LA GRANGE**
LaGrange Nautilus Fitness Center
Dual
Lee's Crossing Shopping Center
Zip Code 30240
Ph. (404) 882-3148

**LITHIA SPRINGS**
Georgia Fitness Center, Inc.
Alt.
3951 Highway 78
Zip Code 30057
Ph. (404) 948-4190

**MARIETTA**
Choi Nautilus   Dual
2719 Canton Road
Zip Code 30066
Ph. (404) 428-7820

Spa Lady Fitness Center –
Women
Parkway Village
1851 Roswell Rd.
Zip Code 30067
Ph. (404) 977-9775

Spa Lady Fitness Center –
Women
South Cobb Village
1983 S. Cobb Dr.
Zip Code 30060
Ph. (404) 432-9415

**MARIETTA – SMURNA**
Nautilus Karate & Fitness Center
Dual
2086 Cobb Pkwy.
Zip Code 30080
Ph. (404) 952-2163

New Life Fitness Centers, Inc.
Dual
2745 Sandy Plains Rd., N.E.
Zip Code 30066
Ph. (404) 973-1700

**NEWNAN**
Nautilus Fitness Club   Dual
P.O. Box 971
18 Bullsboro Dr.
Zip Code 30264
Ph. (404) 253-4437

**NORCROSS**
American Fitness Center   Alt.
5345 Jimmy Carter Blvd.
Zip Code 30093
Ph. (404) 447-8500

Focus on Fitness   Alt.
6135 Peachtree Pkwy.
Zip Code 30092
Ph. (404) 448-4942

**N. AUGUSTA**
Spa Lady Fitness Center
Women
310 E. Martin Town Rd.
North Augusta Plaza
Zip Code 30909
Ph. (404) 738-0635

**ROME**
Kelly Lyn Figure Salons –
Women
No. 4 Gala Shopping Center
Zip Code 30161
Ph. (404) 235-4727

Rome Health Spa – Alt.
28 Central Plaza
Zip Code 30161
Ph. (404) 291-9080

**ROSWELL**
Aerobic Fitness Center and Spa
–Women
599 B Holcomb Bridge Rd.
Zip Code 30075
Ph. (404) 992-5076

Breadaway Fitness Inc. – Women
10516 Alpharetta St.
Zip Code 30075
Ph. (404) 998-2121

**SMYRNA**
American Fitness Center – Alt.
3270 South Cobb Dr.
Zip Code 30080
Ph. (404) 434-8024

**STONE MOUNTAIN**
American Health Fitness Center
– Alt.
5561 Memorial Drive
Zip Code 30083
Ph. (404) 284-9440

Nautilus Fitness Center of Stone
Mountain – Dual
5215 Memorial Dr.
Zip Code 30083
Ph. (404) 296-8143

**VALDOSTA**
Valdosta Health Club – Dual
420 East Northside Drive
Zip Code 31601
Ph. (912) 244-4740

**WARNER ROBINS**
Olympian Village Fitness Center
– Alt.
2050 Watson Boulevard
Zip Code 31093
Ph. (912) 923-8813

# HAWAII

**HONOLULU**
Nautilus Fitness Center – Dual
1314 S. King St.
Zip Code 96814
Ph. (808) 524-7770

**KAILUA**
Natural Man of Kailua – Men
1090 Keolu Drive
Zip Code 96734
Ph. (808) 261-7905

Natural Woman Health & Fitness
Center – Women
116 Hekill
Zip Code 96734
Ph. (808) 261-1796 or 261-1797

# IDAHO

**BOISE**
Lady Fitness – Women
5460 Franklin Rd.
Zip Code 83705
Ph. (203) 344-4366

Family Fitness Center – Alt.
P.O. Box 8506
Zip Code 83704
Ph. (208) 342-8963

**IDAHO FALLS**
Alpha Health Spa   Alt.
1710 East 16th St.
Zip Code 83401
Ph. (208) 522-2712

Alpha Lady   Women
1769 W. Broadway
Zip Code 83401
Ph. (208) 522-2786

**POCATELLO**
Metropolitan Health Spa   Alt.
442 N. Arthur
Zip Code 83201
Ph. (208) 232-4541

**TWIN FALLS**
Sophisticated Lady Fitness Center
Women
226 Eastland Dr.
Zip Code 83301
Ph. (208) 734-7313

# ILLINOIS

**AURORA**
Chicago Health Clubs, Inc. – Dual
4220 Westbrook
Fox Valley Shopping Center
Zip Code 60505
Ph. (313) 898-8700

Lynn Stevens Health Studio –
Women
916 North Farnsworth Ave.
Zip Code 60505
Ph. (312) 851-1331

**BELLEVILLE**
Vic Tanny International   Alt.
700 Carlyle Plaza
Zip Code 62221
Ph. (618) 277-5060

**BLOOMINGDALE**
Nautilus of Bloomingdale    Dual
162 S. Bloomingdale Road
Zip Code 60108
Ph. (317) 351-0707

**BUFFALO GROVE**
Postl Athletic Clubs    Women
1300 W. Dundee
Zip Code 60090
Ph. (312) 259-8438

**CALUMET CITY**
Chicago Health Clubs, Inc.    Dual
1500 S. Torrence Ave.
Zip Code 60409
Ph. (312) 891-8800

**CHICAGO**
Chicago Health Club    Alt.
6451 N. Ridge
Zip Code 60626
Ph. (312) 743-9484

Chicago Health Club    Alt.
4950 W. Fullerton
Zip Code 60639
Ph. (312) 637-9531

Chicago Health Club    Alt.
2038 W. 95th St.
Zip Code 60642
Ph. (312) 233-9799

Nautilus of the Loop, Inc.    Dual
325 N. Wells St.
Zip Code 60610
Ph. (312) 836-9004

Postl Athletic Clubs    Dual
209 W. Jackson
Zip Code 60606
Ph. (312) 922-3049

Postl Athletic Clubs    Dual
188 W. Randolph
Zip Code 60601
Ph. (312) 332-4567

Postl Athletic Clubs    Dual
1050 N. State St.
Zip Code 60601
Ph. (312) 266-9824

**COLLINSVILLE**
American Fitness Center and
Spa    Dual
44 Brink Street
Zip Code 62234
Ph. (618) 344-3330

**CRYSTAL LAKE**
Crystal Lake Nautilus Health
Club    Dual
44 Brink Street
Zip Code 60014
Ph. (815) 459-4030

Lyn Stevens Health Studio
Women
24 Crystal Lake Plaza
Zip Code 60014
Ph. (815) 455-4110

**DANVILLE**
Lyn Stevens Health Studio
Women
2807 North Vermilion
Zip Code 61832
Ph. (217) 443-0353 or 443-0354

**DECATUR**
21st Century Health Spa    Alt.
1700 E. Pershing Rd.
Zip Code 62526
Ph. (217) 877-7570

**DEKALB**
Lyn Stevens Health Studio
Women
205 N. Second Street
Zip Code 60115
Ph. (815) 756-2764

**DIXON**
Lyn Stevens Health Studio –
Women
Pamida Discount Shopping Center
Zip Code 61021
Ph. (815) 284-3347

**DOWNERS GROVE**
Nautilus Health Club – Dual
75th Street & Fairview Ave.
Fairview Plaza
Zip Code 60515
Ph. (312) 969-2199

**ELK GROVE**
Nautilus Fitness Centers – Dual
65 Park-N-SHop
Zip Code 60007
Ph. (312) 439-0700

**ELMHURST**
Nautilus Fitness Centers Inc.
Dual
575 W. St. Charles Rd.
Zip Code 60126
Ph. (312) 530-0100

**FAIRVIEW HEIGHTS**
Vic Tanny International – Alt.
10806 Lincoln Trail
Zip Code 62208
Ph. (618) 398-5914

**FREEPORT**
Lyn Stevens Health Studio –
Women
1803 S. West Ave.

**GRANITE CITY**
Spartan Health & Tennis,
Racquetball Club – Dual
Hwy 111 & 162 at Bradley St.
P.O. Box 691
Zip Code 62040
Ph. (618) 931-2500

**GURNEE**
Nautilus Physical Fitness Center
Dual
811 N. Waveland Ave.
Zip Code 60031
Ph. (312) 662-3111

**HICKORY HILLS**
Nautilus Fitness Center – Dual
8659 W. 95th St.
Zip Code 60457
Ph. (312) 598-3313

**HIGHLAND**
Fitness Now – Alt.
Northtown Shopping Center
Zip Code 62249
Ph. (618) 654-7585

**HIGHLAND PARK**
Chicago Health Clubs – Alt.
Crossroad Shopping Center
Clavey Rd. and Edens Expressway
Zip Code 60035
Ph. (312) 831-9847

**KANKAKEE**
Surf Side Health Club    Dual
Route 49-52 South
P.O. Box 205
Zip Code 60901
Ph. (815) 935-2100

Woman's World Health and Fitness Center    Women
221 S. Schuyler
Zip Code 60901
Ph. (815) 937-1911

**LaGRANGE**
Chicago Health Club    Alt.
35 La Grange Rd.
Zip Code 60625
Ph. (312) 352-9776

**LIBERTYVILLE**
Nautilus Fitness Club    Dual
850 S. Milwaukee Ave.
Zip Code 60048
Ph. (312) 680-7040

**LOMBARD**
Chicago Health & Racquet Club
Dual
455 E. Butterfield Rd.
Zip Code 60142
Ph. (312) 963-3600

**MARION**
Cleopatra Health Spa – Women
Westmore Plaza
Zip Code 62959
Ph. (618) 997-6359

**MATTESON**
Chicago Health Clubs, Inc.    Dual
4701 Lincoln Mall
Zip Code 60443
Ph. (312) 481-9191

**MORTON GROVE**
Chicago Health Club    Alt.
5835 Dempster
Zip Code 60053
Ph. (312) 967-9191

**MOUNT PROSPECT**
Chicago Health Club    Alt.
225 West Rand St.
Zip Code 60056
Ph. (312) 253-9830

**MUNDELEIN**
Lyn Stevens Health Studio
Women
372 Townline Road
Zip Code 60060
Ph. (312) 566-1880

**MT. ZION**
21st Century Health Spa    Alt.
2048 Mt. Zion
Zip Code 62549
Ph. (217) 429-0671

**NAPERVILLE**
Lyn Stevens Health Studio
Women
140 W. Gartner Rd.
Zip Code 60504
Ph. (312) 357-7171

Nautilus Mind and Body Fitness
Center   Dual
1458 E. Chicago Ave.
Zip Code 60450
Ph. (312) 420-1600

NILES
Nautilus Fitness Center   Dual
8273 Golf
Zip Code 60648
Ph. (312) 967-0333

Postl Atletic Clubs   Women
7900 N. Milwaukee
Zip Code 60648
Ph. (312) 965-1033

OAK BROOK
Chicago Health Clubs   Fair
Lady, Inc.   Women
30 Oak Brook Mall
Zip Code 60521
Ph. (312) 654-0868

OAK LAWN
Chicago Health Clubs, Inc.   Dual
6700 West 95th St.
Zip Code 60453
Ph. (312) 439-3500

OAK PARK
Chicago Health Club   Alt.
345 Madison St.
Zip Code 60302
Ph. (312) 383-9835

ORLAND PARK
Chicago Health Clubs, Inc.   Dual
147th and LaGrange Road
Zip Code 60462
Ph. (312) 349-0100

Nautilus Physical Fitness &
Racquetball Center   Dual
16545 S. 71st Ct.
Zip Code 60462
Ph. (312) 532-0088

PALATINE
Nautilus Conditioning Center
Dual
807 E. Dundee
Zip Code 60067
Ph. (312) 359-3760

PARKRIDGE
Chicago Health Clubs   Fair
Lady, Inc.   Women
626 Talcott Road
Zip Code 60068
Ph. (312) 696-4444

PEORIA
Nucleus Health Club   Dual
3024 West Lake Ave.
Zip Code 61614
Ph. (309) 682-0821

RANTOUL
Nautilus Health Spa, Inc. - Alt.
8939 East 38th
Northeast Wood Chopping Center
Zip Code 46226
Ph. (317) 898-6115

Olympia Lady Spa Fitness Center
—Women
3812 H. High School Rd.
Zip Code 46254
Ph. (317) 298-8188

Olympia Lady Spa Fitness Center
—Women
9415 N. Meridian St.
Zip Code 46260
Ph. (317) 848-1417

Olympia Lady Spa Fitness Center
- Women
9727 E. Washington St.
Zip Code 46229
Ph. (317) 899-2550

Olympic Super Spa – Dual
6020 Crawfordsville Rd.
Zip Code 46224
Ph. (317) 247-9100

Silhouette National Health Spa
- Alt.
7325 West 10th Street
Zip Code 46224
Ph. (317) 271-6837

Silhouette National Health Spa
- Alt.
8085 South Madison Ave.
Zip Code 46227
Ph. (317) 888-7211

Silhouette National Health Spa
Alt.
7216 North Keystone Ave.
Zip Code 46240
Ph. (317) 257-1489

Silhouette National Health Spa
- Alt.
6407 East Washington St.
Zip Code 46219
Ph. (317) 356-7223

Speedway Health Spa – Alt.
4575 W. 16th St.
Zip Code 46224
Ph. (317) 243-6630

Lyn Stevens Health Studio –
Women
Rantoul Plaza
Hwy 136 East
Zip Code 62866
Ph. (217) 893-8806

RICHTON PARK
Olympic Fitness – Dual
3728 W. Sauk Trail
Zip Code 60471
Ph. (312) 748-7580

ROCKFORD
Nautilus Fitness Center – Dual
3929 Broadway
Zip Code 61108
Ph. (815) 226-0403

Rockford Health and Racquet
Club   Alt.
3800 E. State St.
Zip Code 61108
Ph. (815) 398-8293

ST. CHARLES
Lyn Stevens Health Studios
Women
1515 W. Main St.
Zip Code 60174
Ph. (312) 232-6116

SCHAUMBURG
Chicago Health & Tennis Club
Dual
1020 Meacham Rd.
Zip Code 60172
Ph. (312) 885-0800

Postl Athletic Clubs   Women
833 West Higgins
Zip Code 60195
Ph. (312) 843-1770

SKOKIE
Chicago Health Clubs, Fair Lady,
Inc.   Women
64 Old Orchard Road
Zip Code 60076
Ph. (312) 674-9600

SOUTH HOLLAND
Nautilus Fitness Center   Dual
16250 Prince Drive
Zip Code 60473
Ph. (312) 331-3993

SPRINGFIELD
Silhouette Figure Form – Alt.
3137 S. Dirksen Pkwy.
Capital City Shopping Center
Zip Code 62703
Ph. (217) 529-0400

Silhouette American Health Spa
- Alt.
1650 Wabash   The Yard
Zip Code 62704
Ph. (217) 546-6707 or 793-0016

SYCAMORE
Olympic Health & Racquet Club
Dual
2496 DeKalb Ave.
Zip Code 60178
Ph. (815) 756-6381

TAYLORVILLE
World of Health   Alt.
105 East Bidwell
Zip Code 62568
Ph. (217) 278-7261

VERNON HILLS
Fair Lady, Inc.   Women
30 Philip Road (at Rte 60)
Zip Code 60060
Ph. (312) 680-3000

WAUKEGAN
Spa Fitness Center   Alt.
1900 Belvedere
Zip Code 60085
Ph. (312) 336-6330

WHEATON
Postl Athletic Clubs   Dual
1 Wheaton Center
Zip Code 60187
Ph. (312) 653-2040

WHEELING
Nautilus Exercenters   Dual
471 E. Dundee Rd.
Zip Code 60090
Ph. (312) 541-8400

WOODRIVER
Spartan Health Club   Dual
48 E. Ferguson
Zip Code 62095
Ph. (618) 254-3861

## INDIANA

**ANDERSON**
Olympic Spas, Inc.    Alt.
2709 Nichol Ave.
Zip Code 46011
Ph. (317) 649-5564

**BEECH GROVE**
Olympia Lady Spa Fitness Center
   Women
323 S. 1st Street
Zip Code 46107
Ph. (317) 787-3225

**BLOOMINGTON**
Barzo's Nautilus Fitness Center
   Dual
Curry Pike/Highland Village
Zip Code 47401
Ph. (812) 339-8235

**BRAZIL**
Nautilus Family Fitness Center
   Dual
20 S. Lambert St.
Zip Code 47834
Ph. (812) 442-1282

**CARMEL**
Carmel Family Health Spa    Alt
622 South Range Line Rd.
Zip Code 46032
Ph. (317) 844-6396

**CLARKSVILLE**
Holiday Spa    Alt.
1590 Greentree Blvd.
Zip Code 47130
Ph. (812) 288-9263

**COLUMBUS**
Supreme Health Spa    Alt.
2321 Marr Road
Zip Code 47201
Ph. (812) 372-9963

**CRAWFORDSVILLE**
Right Weight Family Fitness
   Centre    Alt.
407 E. Market Street
Zip Code 47933
Ph. (317) 362-0986

**ELKHART**
New Era Health Club    Dual
1112 W. Bristol
Zip Code 46514
Ph. (219) 264-4113

**EVANSVILLE**
My Fair Lady Spa, Inc.    Women
3411 1st Ave.
Zip Code 47710
Ph. (812) 426-2717

My Fair Lady Spa, Inc.    Women
4820 Tecumseh Land
Zip Code 47715
Ph. (812) 477-6451

21st Century Health Spa    Alt.
4920 Bellemeade Ave.
Zip Code 47715
Ph. (812) 479-0267

**FORT WAYNE**
american Health Fitness Centers
   Alt.
4810 North Clinton St.
Zip Code 46805
Ph. (219) 484-2657

American Health Fitness Centers
   Alt.
6810 U.S. Hwy. 27, South
Zip Code 46816
Ph. (219) 447-1566

**FRANKLIN**
Franklin Health Club    Alt.
152 E. Jefferson St.
Zip Code 46131
Ph. (317) 736-8888

**INDIANAPOLIS**
Nautilus Executive Fitness Center
   Men
20 North Meridian
Zip Code 46204
Ph. (317) 631-9977

Nautilus Health Spas    Alt.
4702 Century Plaza Rd.
Zip Code 46254
Ph. (317) 298-9810

Nautilus Health Spa, Inc.    Dual
4702 Century Plaza Road
Zip Code 46254
Ph. (317) 298-9810

**KOKOMO**
New Life Health Spa – Alt.
1951 S. Elizabeth
Zip Code 46901
Ph. (317) 457-6651

**MARION**
Nautilus Health & Fitness Center
   – Dual
714 South Adams St.
Zip Code 46952
Ph. (317) 662-9977

**MERRILLVILLE**
Nautilus Fitness Center    Dual
1205 West Lincoln Highway
Zip Code 46410
Ph. (219) 769-7117

**MUNCIE**
Silhouette National Health Spa
   Alt.
4613 North Wheeling Ave.
Zip Code 47304
Ph. (317) 289-7958

**NEW CASTLE**
New Life Fitness Center    Alt.
510 S. Memorial
Zip Code 47362
Ph. (317) 521-3010

**RICHMOND**
New Life Health Spa    Alt.
4714 National Rd. East
Zip Code 47374
Ph. (317) 966-2516

**SHELBYVILLE**
Regal International Health Spa
   Dual
2712 East St. Rd. 44
Zip Code 46176
Ph. (317) 398-0165

**SOUTH BEND**
Spa Fitness Center    Alt.
3703 N. Main
   Mishawaka
Zip Code 46544
Ph. (219) 255-3101

**WEST LAFAYETTE**
Dean's Family Fitness Center
   Alt.
360 Brown Street 'evee
Zip Code 47906
Ph. (317) 743-4657

## IOWA

**AMES**
Brunia's Physical Conditioning
   Center    Dual
1619 S.E. High St.
Zip Code 50010
Ph. (515) 233-3521

**CEDAR RAPIDS**
King Richard's Fitness Center
   Alt.
222 Glenbrook Drive, S.E.
Zip Code 52403
Ph. (319) 393-8710

**CORALVILLE**
Royale Health Centre    Dual
704 First Avenue
Cantebury Inn Motel
Zip Code 52241
Ph. (319) 351-5577

**DES MOINES**
Des Moines Athletic Center
   Men
1120 Walnut
Zip Code 50309
Ph. (515) 284-8990

Kim's Academy (East)    Dual
2956 E. University
Zip Code 50317
Ph. (515) 263-1101

Kim's Academy Nautilus Fitness
   Dual
7560 Hickman Rd.
Zip Code 50322
Ph. (515) 270-1600

Kim's Nautilus Gym Center, Inc.
4626 S.W. 9th St., Suite 800
Zip Code 50315
Ph. (515) 287-6898

New Image Family Fitness Center
   Dual
3520 Beaver Avenue, Suite D
Zip Code 50310
Ph. (515) 277-0268

**DUBUQUE**
Century Health Club    Dual
805 Century Drive
Century Plaza
Zip Code 52001
Ph. (319) 583-8256 or 556-9430

**MUSCATINE**
Royal Spa & Health Center    Alt.
2402 Park Avenue
Zip Code 52761
Ph. (319) 264-1221

**SIOUX CITY**
Kim's Nautilus Fitness Center
   Dual
1551 Indian Hills Dr., No. 106
Zip Code 51104
Ph. (712) 252-3832

Morningside Fitness Center   Alt.
1819 Morningside Ave.
Zip Code 51106
Ph. (712) 276-6541

## KANSAS

EMPORIA
Magic Mirror Figure Salons
Women
1400 Industrial Rd.
Zip Code 66801
Ph. (316) 343-7950

KANSAS CITY
Indian Springs Fitness Center
Dual
Indian Springs Shopping Center
4601 State Ave.
Zip Code 66102
Ph. (913) 287-3110

LAWRENCE
Magic Mirror Figure Salons
Women
601 Kasoid Dr., C-107
Zip Code 66044

MANHATTAN
Nautilus Fitness Center of Man-
hattan   Dual
1122 Laramie
Zip Code 66502
Ph. (913) 776-1654

TOPEKA
American Health & Fitness of
Topeka   Women
1501 W. 21st
Zip Code 66604
Ph. (913) 354-7721

**Sun Yi's TKD Nautilus Fitness
Center — Dual
921 W. 37th St.
Zip Code 66609
Ph. (913) 266-5974**

WICHITA
Mademoiselle Spa -- Women
6100 E. Central Ave.
Zip Code 67208
Ph. (316) 688-5616

Nautilus of Wichita — Dual
3940 W. Douglas
Zip Code 67203
Ph. (316) 823-0176

Win's Super Fitness World — Dual
2234 S. Oliver
Zip Code 67218
Ph. (316) 682-1573

Win's Super Fitness World — Dual
777 N. West Street
Zip Code 67203
Ph. (316) 942-3237

## KENTUCKY

ASHLAND
She Figure & Fitness Spa —
Women
2818 Moore St.
Zip Code 41101
Ph. (606) 329-9971

BOWLING GREEN
Imperial Health Spas, Inc.   Alt.
1901 Russelville Rd.
Western Gateway Shopping
Center
Zip Code 42101
Ph. (502) 781-1151

FLORENCE
Future Fitness by Nautilus   Dual
8415 U.S. 42
Zip Code 41042
Ph. (606) 525-8886

FRANKFORT
She Figure & Fitness Spa —
Women
1230 U.S. 127 South
Zip Code 40601
Ph. (502) 223-0522

FT. WRIGHT
Spa Lady — Women
1981 Dixie Hwy.
Zip Code 41011
Ph. (606) 341-0812

GLASGOW
The Fitness Center — Alt.
Parkview Shopping Center
Park Ave. next to Houchen's
Zip Code 42141
Ph. (502) 651-2911

HOPKINSVILLE
Pennyrile Racquetball I Health
Club   Dual
104 Bradshaw Pike Ext.
Zip Code 42240
Ph. (502) 885-4200

LEXINGTON
My Fair Lady Spa   Women
157 Eastland Shopping Ctr.
Ph. (606) 252-6718

My Fair Lady Spa   Women
197 Moore Dr.
Zip Code 40503
Ph. (606) 276-3580

My Fair Lady Spa   Women
North Park Shopping Ctr.
Ph. (606) 265-8059

21st Century Health Spa   Alt.
1077 S. Broadway
Zip Code 40504
Ph. (606) 255-6827

21st Century Health Spa   Alt.
2683 Regency Road
Zip Code 40503
Ph. (606) 278-9328

LOUISVILLE
Holiday Spa   Alt.
7100 Preston Highway
Zip Code 40219
Ph. (502) 966-5241

Holiday Spa   Alt.
3934 Dixie Hwy.
Zip Code 40216
Ph. (502) 448-3211

Holiday Spa — Dual
9070 Dixie Hwy.
Zip Code 40258
Ph. (502) 935-4053

MADISONVILLE
Total Fitness Inc.   Women
Madison Square Shopping Center
Zip Code 42431
Ph. (502) 821-0326

NEWPORT
Forum Health Spa   Alt.
68 Carothers Rd.
Newport Plaza Shopping Center
Zip Code 41071
Ph. (606) 292-0166

OWENSBORO
Athenian Spa Inc.   Alt.
4026 Fredrica St.
Zip Code 42301
Ph. (502) 684-1495

FT. WRIGHT
Spa Lady   Women
1981 Dixie Hwy.
Zip Code 41011
Ph. (606) 341-0812

## LOUISIANA

ALEXANDRIA
The Health Spa   Alt.
1020 MacArthur Drive
Zip Code 71301
Ph. (318) 445-6496

Kelly Lyn Figure Salons
Women
1305 Metro Dr.
Zip Code 71391
Ph. (318) 473-0322

BATON ROUGE
All American Health Spa   Dual
8889 Sullivan Rd.
Zip Code 70805
Ph. (504) 261-8372

Cosmopolitan Lady   Women
11135 Florida Ave.
Zip Code 70815
Ph. (504) 273-3030

Foxy's Health Club   Alt.
4343 Rhoda Dr.
Zip Code 70816
Ph. (504) 293-9860

Kelly Lyn Figure Salons
Women
Corporate Mall
5280-88 Corporate Blvd.
Zip Code 70808
Ph. (504) 927-9001

Kelly Lyn Figure Salons
Women
Bell Aire Plaza
12131 Florida Blvd.
Zip Code 70815
Ph. (504) 272-5830

Olympia Health Spa — Dual
3032 College Dr.
Zip Code 70808
Ph. (504) 924-5327

BOSSIER CITY
Fountain of Youth Health Resort
Dual
3515 East Texas.
Zip Code 71111
Ph. (318) 742-6337

World Wide Health Studios
Dual
108 Bossier Center
Zip Code 71111
Ph. (318) 746-0474

GRETNA
Nautilus Health Center    Dual
2007 Daniels Rd.
Zip Code 70053
Ph. (504) 366-8161

HARAHAN
Aquarius Health Spa    Dual
1192 S. Clearview Parkway
Zip Code 70123
Ph. (504) 733-7721

KAPLAN
Olympus Fitness Resort    Dual
Hwy. 14 East
Zip Code 70548
Ph. (318) 643-6069

KENNER
Lady Fitness    Women
2460 Veterans Blvd.
Zip Code 70062
Py. (504) 469-3433

LAFAYETTE
Fitness Resort, Inc. — Dual
333 Frontage Road
Zip Code 70502
Ph. (318) 234-3263

LAKE CHARLES
Dave's Swedish Spa — Alt.
2129 Oak Park Boulevard
Zip Code 70601
Ph. (318) 478-7300

Roman Spa, Nautilus & Racquetball Club — Dual
4324 Lake Street
Zip Code 70605
Ph. (318) 478-8510

LAPLACE
LaPlace Health Club — Dual
518 Hemlock St.
Zip Code 70068
Ph. (504) 652-1399

MARRERO
Grecian Health Spa
857 Avenue C
Zip Code 70072
Ph. (504) 347-9423

METAIRE
Jefferson Parish Health Club —
Co-ed
3225 Danny Pk.
Zip Code 70002
Ph. (504) 885-6200

Lakeside Health Club — Men
3414 Hessmer Ave.
Zip Code 70002
Ph. (504) 888-2033

MONROE
Kelly Lyn Figure Salons
Women
1613 N. 18th St.
Murray Place Shopping Center
Zip Code 71201
Ph. (318) 388-3232

NEW IBERIA
Cypress Health Club — Alt.
1800 E. Main St.
Zip Code 70560
Ph. (318) 367-1576

Romana Figure Spa — Women
173 Duperior
Zip Code 70560
Ph. (318) 365-1408

NEW ORLEANS
Nautilus Health Center — Dual
921 Canal St., 6th floor
Zip Code 70112
Ph. (504) 542-2287

PLAQUEMINE
Isokinetic Fitness Center — Alt.
414 La Bauve Ave.
Zip Code 70764
Ph. (504) 687-2011

SHREVEPORT
Louisa Health & Beauty Resort
Women
1935 E. 70th St.
Zip Code 71105
Ph. (318) 797-7000

Louisa Health & Beauty Resort
Women
2920 Truly Lane
Zip Code 71118
Ph. (318) 687-1442

Nautilus Fitness Center — Alt.
990 Quail Creek Rd.
Zip Code 71105
Ph. (318) 865-3579

World Wide Health Studios
Dual
4048 Youree Dr.
Zip Code 71105
Ph. (318) 865-1444

World Wide Health Studios
Dual
2738 Mackey Lane
Zip Code 71108
Ph. (318) 686-1606

SULPHUR
Roman Spa & Nautilus Club
Alt.
918 Post Oak Road
Zip Code 70601
Ph. (318) 625-4232

# MAINE

BIDDEFORD
Woman's World Health Spa —
Women
335 Alfred St.
Zip Code 04005
Ph. (207) 283-0131

PORTLAND
Woman's World Health Spa —
Women
91 Auburn St.
Zip Code 04103
Ph. (207) 797-0446 or 0447

SPRINGVALE
Figure Magic Health Spa
Women
Shopper's Square, Bridge Street
Zip Code 04083
Ph. (207) 324-0482

# MARYLAND

ANNAPOLIS
Nautilus Annapolis    Dual
1981 MOreland Pkwy.
Zip Code 21401
Ph. (301) 267-0515

BALTIMORE
Future Shapes of Putty Hill
Women
Putty Hill Plaza
7956 Belair Road
Zip Code 21236
Ph. (301) 661-4870

Metro Nautilus Fitness Centers
Dual
1 E. Chase St.
Zip Code 21202
Ph. (301) 727-5151

Nautilus Security Total Fitness
Center    Dual
2076 Lord Baltimore Dr.
Zip Code 21207
Ph. (301) 298-1300

Riviera Health Spa
6638 Security Blvd.
Zip Code 21207
Ph. (301) 944-9177

BOWIE
Witemarsh Racquet & Country
Club Fitness Center — Dual
Whitemarsh Park Drive
Zip Code 27015
Ph. (301) 262-4553

CAMP SPRINGS
Fun & Fitness — Dual
Allentown Mall
6278 Branch Ave.
Zip Code 20023
Ph. (301) 449-3262

CLINTON
Contemporary Woman Figure Spa
— Women
Clinton Park Shopping Center
8807 Woodyard Rd.
Zip Code 20735
Ph. (301) 868-8870

COCKEYSVILLE
Modern Woman Figure Salon —
Women
33 Cranbrook Rd.
Zip Code 21030
Ph. (301) 628-7590

DUNDALK
Metro Nautilus Fitness Centers —
Dual
6400 Beckley
Zip Code 21222
Ph. (301) 633-8600

EASTON
Future Shapes of Easton
Easton Plaza
Zip Code 21601
Ph. (301) 822-8881

FREDERICK
Future Shapes of Frederick —
Women
Frederick Towne Mall
Route 40
Zip Code 21701
Ph. (301) 694-9393

GAITHERSBURG
Future Shapes of Gaithersburg —
Women
501 N. Frederick
Zip Code 20760
Ph. (301) 258-0542

Spa Lady — Women
230 N. Frederick
Zip Code 20760
Ph. (301) 926-2910

GREENBELT
Looking Good — Women
6176 Greenbelt Rd.
Beltway Plaza
Zip Code 20770
Ph. (301) 474-5544

HAGERSTOWN
Apollo-Dianna Health Spa — Alt.
1350 Dual Highway
Zip Code 21740
Ph. (301) 797-4700

Future Shapes — Women
Valley Plaza
Zip Code 21740

JOPPA
Future Shapes of Joppa — Women
1012 Joppa Farm Rd.
Zip Code 21085
Ph. (301) 679-6880

LUTHERVILLE
Metro Nautilus Fitness Centers —
Dual
Falls & Valley Roads
Zip Code 21093
Ph. (301) 337-9500

NEW CARROLLTON
Heartbeat Figure Salon — Women
7560 Riverdale Rd.
Zip Code 20764
Ph. (301) 459-7280

OWINGS MILLS
Metro Nautilus Fitness Centers —
Dual
66 Painters Mill Rd.
Zip Code 21117
Ph. (301) 363-4988

ODENTON
Bodies-in-Motion — Women
417 B Telegraph Rd.
Zip Code 21113
Ph. (301) 674-4666

PASADENA
Bodies-in-Motion — Women
8176 Jumpers Mall
Zip Code 21122
Ph. (301) 787-0404

PIKESVILLE
Nautilus at the Hilton — Dual
Reisterstown Rd. at the Beltway
Zip Code 21208
Ph. (301) 486-2606

REISTERSTOWN
The Body Factory — Alt.
Chartley Shopping Center
144-A Chartley Drive
Zip Code 21136
Ph. (301) 833-2024

ROCKVILLE
Chuck Foreman's Nautilus Fitness
Center — Dual
38 Courthouse Square
Zip Code 20850
Ph. (301) 762-1970

Fitness World — Women
1691 Rockville Pike
Zip Code 20852
Ph. (301) 770-6930

Spa Lady — Women
1776 E. Jefferson St.
Zip Code 20852
Ph. (301) 881-7333

Total Woman, Otd. — Women
2003 Viers Mill Road
Zip Code 20852
Ph. (301) 279-2660

SALISBURY
Nautilus of Salisbury
201 Milford St.
Zip Code 21801
Ph. (301) 546-5731

SEVERNA PARK
Metro Nautilus — Dual
1902 Ritchie Hwy.
Zip Code 21012
Ph. (301) 544-2525

SUITLAND
Fun & Fitness, Inc. — Dual
Silver Hill Plaza
5836 Silver Hill Rd.
Zip Code 20023
Ph. (301) 420-5100

TEMPLE HILLS
Fun & Fitness of Rosecroft —
Men
3245 Brinkley Rd.
Rosecroft Shopping Ctr.
Zip Code 20031
Ph. (301) 894-4600

TOWSON
Grecian Lady Figure Salon —
Women
6831 Loch Raven Blvd.
Hillen Dale Shopping Center
Zip Code 21234
Ph. (301) 321-6647

Metro Nautilus Fitness Center —
Dual
8757 Mylander Lane
Zip Code 21204
Ph. (301) 321-0081

WALDORF
St. Charles Fitness Center — Dual
Smallwood Village Center
Zip Code 20601
Ph. (301) 843-1234

WESTMINISTER
Leisure Health Spa — Alt.
425 Manchester Rd.
Zip Code 21157
Ph. (301) 848-2020

## MASSACHUSETTS

ACTON
Woman's World Health & Figure
Salon — Women
202 Nagog Square (Route 2-A)
Zip Code 01720
Ph. (617) 263-2921

ANDOVER
Rolling Green Health & Fitness
Center — Dual
193 & Rt. 133
Zip Code 01810
Ph. (617) 475-0438

Woman's World Health Spas —
Women
90 Main Street
Zip Code 01810
Ph. (617) 475-7840

BOSTON
Presidents-Forst Lady Spa — Alt.
715 Granite St.
Braintree
Zip Code 02184
Ph. (617) 848-3345

Presidents-First Lady Spa — Alt.
575 Worcester
Framingham
Zip Code 01701
Ph. (617) 872-4815

BOURNE
Modern Woman Figure Salon, Inc.
— Women
160 Mac Arthur Blvd.
Zip Code 02532
Ph. (617) 759-4994

BOXBORO
Boxboro Health & Recreation
Club — Alt.
242 Sheraton Rd.
Zip Code 01719
Ph. (617) 263-3967

BRAINTREE
Woman's World Health Spa —
Women
400 Franklin Street
Zip Code 02184
Ph. (617) 843-8383

BROOKLINE
Woman's World Health Spa —
Women
62R Harvard St.
Zip Code 02146
Ph. 232-7440

BROCKTON
Woman's World Health Spa —
Women
Westgate Plaza
Zip Code 02401
Ph. (617) 588-1818

BURLINGTON
World of Health Spa — Dual
Cambridge Street
Exit 41 — Burlington Plaza
Zip Code 01803
Ph. (617) 272-3060

Woman's World Health Spas —
Women
Westgate Shopping Center
Intersection of Rt. 495 & Rt. 110
Zip Code 01830
Ph. (617) 373-1297

Woman's World Health Spas —
Women
Plaza 62
85 Wilmington Rd.
Zip Code 01803
Ph. (617) 273-0418

CAMBRIDGE
Woman's World Health Spa —
Women
2000 Aassachusetts Ave., Orter
Square
Zip Code 02140
Ph. (617) 491-3707

CANTON
Woman's World Health Spa —
Women
95 Washington St.
Zip Code 02021
Ph. (617) 828-8640

CHELMSFORD
Women's World Health Spa &
Figure Salon — Women
29-31 Summer St.
"The Market Place"
Zip Code 01824
Ph. (617) 256-8916

DANVERS
Woman's World Health Spa —
Women
Endicott Plaza, Endicott St.
Zip Code 01923
Ph. (617) 774-0223

EAST LONGMEADOW
Meadow's East Health Club —
Dual
18 Benjamin Street
Zip Code 01028
Ph. (413) 525-6628

EAST MILTON
Woman's World Health Spa —
Women
364 Granite Ave.
Zip Code 02186
Ph. (617) 698-0260

FRAMINGHAM
Roman Health Spa Racquetball —
Dual
61 Nicholas Road
Zip Code 01701
Ph. (617) 877-1857

Woman's World Health Spas —
Women
Deerskin Plaza
680 Worcester Rd.
Zip Code 01701
Ph. (617) 620-1363

World of Health Spas — Dual
855 Worcester Rd.
Route 9, Trolley Square
Zip Code 01701
Py. (617) 875-6148

FRANKLIN
Woman's World Health Spa —
Women
Franklin Shoppers Fair
254 E. Central St.
Zip Code 02038
Ph. (617) 528-7300

GREENFIELD
Cherry Rum Health Spa —
Women
493 Bernardston Road
Zip Code 01301
Ph. (413) 774-2275

HANOVER
World of Health Spa — Dual
No. 1 Washington St.
Route 3 Exit 31 — Hanover Mall
Zip Code 02339
Ph. (617) 826-8351

Woman's World Health Spa —
Women
Hanover Shopping Center
Route 53
Zip Code 02339
Ph. (617) 826-2366

HAVERHILL
Woman's World    Women
Westgate Plaza
Zip Code 01830
Ph. (617) 688-9020

HINGHAM
Woman's World Health Spa &
Figure Salon
400 Lincoln St.
(rt. 3A), Lincoln Plaza
Zip Code 02043
Ph. (617) 749-3225

LEOMINSTER
Feel Fit Health Center — Women
Twin City Mall
Zip Code 01453
Ph. (617) 534-1000

LYNN
Joy Health Spa — Women
254 Western Ave.
Zip Code 01904
Ph. (617) 599-4201

LYNNFIELD
House of Health — Dual
379 Broadway — Route 1
Zip Code 01940
Ph. (617) 598-3950

MALDEN
Polaris — Dual
67 Exchange St.
Zip Code 02148
Ph. (617) 395-8516

Woman's World — Women
345 Pleasant St.
Zip Code 02148
Ph. (617) 324-2185

MANSFIELD
Mansfield Health, Fitness &
Racquetball Center — Dual
31 Hampshire St.
Zip Code 02048
Ph. (617) 339-9571

MARLBORO
Woman's World Health Spa —
Women
331 boston Post Rd.
Zip Code 02048
Ph. (617) 481-2005

MEDFORD
Woman's World Fitness Center —
Women
682 Fellsway Shopping Plaza
Zip Code 02155
Ph. (617) 391-2751

MEDFORD SQUARE
Universal Fitness Center — Dual
12 High St.
Zip Code 02155
Ph. (617) 395-4130

MELROSE
Joy Health Spa — Women
39 W. Foster St.
Zip Code 02176
Ph. (617) 391-2751

NATICK
Obie's Exercise Center — Alt.
Hilton Inn, Speen St.
Zip Code 01760
Ph. (617) 653-6825

NEWTON
Woman's World Health Spa —
Women
Marshall's Shopping Center
281 Needham St.
Zip Code 02162
Ph. (617) 964-5136

NORWOOD
Woman's World — Women
428 Walpole St. Route 1A
Norwood King Plaza
Zip Code 02062
Ph. (617) 769-4646

PEABODY
World of Health Spas — Dual
Holiday Inn
1 Newberry St.
Zip Code 01960
Ph. (617) 535-5590

RANDOLPH
Joy Health Spa — Women
1395 N. Main St.
Zip Code 02368
Ph. (617) 963-0349

RAYNHAM
Woman's World Health Spas —
Women
K-Mart Center
Rts. 44 & 24 (South St.)
Zip Code 02767
Ph. (617) 823-4944

READING
Universal Fitness Centre of
Reading — Men
349 Main St.
Zip Code 01867
Ph. (617) 944-4020

**SALEM**
Woman's World Health Spas —
Women
Hawthorne Square Shopping
Center
227 Highland Ave.
Zip Code 01970
Ph. (617) 744-1814 or 1942

**SAUGUS**
Woman's World Health Spa —
Women
Augustine's Plaza
Zip Code 01906
Ph. (617) 233-3112

**SOMERSET**
Woman's World Fitness Center
Somerset Plaza, G.A.R. Hwy.
Zip Code 02725
Ph. (617) 675-0119 or 675-0110

**SOUTH WEYMOUTH**
Woman's World Health Spa —
Women
Pleasant Shopping Center
Route 18
Zip Code 02190
Ph. (617) 331-1206

**SPRINGFIELD**
The Athletic Club & Health
Centre — Men
1203 Parker Street (16 Acres)
Zip Code 01129
Ph. (413) 782-0165

**TEWKSBURY**
Fitness Plus Health Center —
Women
1900 Main St.
Zip Code 01876
Ph. (617) 851-5929

**WALTHAM**
Woman's World — Women
350 Moody St.
Zip Code 02154
Ph. (617) 891-9070

World of Health Spas — Alt.
564 Main St.
Zip Code 02154
Ph. (617) 894-3534

**WATERTOWN**
Woman's World Health Spa —
Women
210 Dexter Ave.
Zip Code 02171
Ph. (617) 926-6262

**WEST BOYLSTON**
Woman's World Health Spas —
Women
W. Boylston Plaza
W. Boylston St. (Rt. 12)
Zip Code 01583
Ph. (617) 835-6242 or 835-6243

**WEST BRIDGEWATER**
Woman's World Health Spa
South Shopping Center
N. Main Street
Zip Code 02379
Ph. (617) 586-1600

**WESTWOOD**
Woman's World Health Spa —
Women
Lamberts 128 Plaza
Providence Hwy.
Zip Code 02090
Ph. (617) 329-1357

**WORCESTER**
International Health Club — Alt.
Lincoln Plaza
535 Lincoln St.
Zip Code 01605
Ph. (617) 852-3813

# MICHIGAN

**ANN ARBOR**
Vic Tanny International — Dual
3860 Washtenaw
Zip Code 48104
Ph. (313) 434-5000

**BATTLE CREEK**
Battle Creek Health Club — Dual
582-588 Capital Ave., SW
Zip Code 48015
Ph. (616) 963-6046

**BAY CITY**
Olympic Health World — Dual
2950 Center Road
Zip Code 48732
Ph. (517) 892-8591

**BIRMINGHAM**
Vic Tanny International — Alt.
625 South Hunter
Zip Code 48011
Ph. (313) 647-5800

**CANTON**
Total Health Spa Inc. of Canton
— Women
45168 Ford Road
Zip Code 48187
Ph. (313) 459-4040

**DEARBORN**
Vic Tanny International — Dual
22324 Michigan Ave.
Zip Code 48124
Ph. (313) 561-3320

**FARMINGTON HILLS**
Nautilus Fitness Center — Dual
28350 W. 8 Mile
Zip Code 48024
Ph. (313) 476-7118

**FLINT**
Vic Tanny Health & Racquet
Club — Dual
4141 Miller Road
Zip Code 48507
Ph. (313) 733-5340

**GRAND RAPIDS**
American Health Fitness Center
Alt.
2755 Birchcrest, S.E.
Zip Code 49506
Ph. (616) 942-0100

American Health Fitness Center
Dual
3470 Plainfield Ave. N.E.
Zip Code 49505
Ph. (616) 364-8731

American Health Fitness Center
— Alt.
2828 28th Street S.W.
Wyoming
Zip Code 49418
Ph. (616) 538-4270

**GROSSE POINT WOODS**
Vic Tanny International — Alt.
20835 Mack Ave.
Zip Code 48236
Ph. (313) 881-6161

**JACKSON**
American Health Fitness Center
— Alt.
2020 Clinton Road
Zip Code 49202
Ph. (517) 787-9292

**KALAMAZOO**
American Health Fitness Center
— Dual
2839 W. Main
Zip Code 49007
Ph. (616) 343-1274

Kalamazoo Center Health Club
— Dual
100 W. Michigan Ave.
Zip Code 49007
Ph. (616) 381-5390

**LIVONIA**
Family Fitness Center
33505 W. 8 Mile
Zip Code 48152
Ph. (313) 371-4482

Vic Tanny International — Alt.
29220 Seven Mile Road
Zip Code 48152
Ph. (313) 476-1314

**MADISON HEIGHTS**
Lady Nautilus, Inc. — Women
30683 Dequindre
Zip Code 48071
Ph. (313) 585-6136

Biofit Systems — Men
30701 Dequindre
Zip Code 48071
Ph. (313) 585-7363

**MIDLAND**
Valley Health World of Midland
— Alt.
2525 Washington
Zip Code 48640
Ph. (517) 631-8800

**MONROE**
Vic Tanny International — Alt.
15266 S. Monroe St.
Zip Code 48161
Ph. (313) 242-0924

**MUSKEGON**
American Health Fitness Center
— Alt.
100 Seaway Drive
Muskegon Heights
Zip Code 49444
Ph. (616) 739-9489

**OAK PARK**
Vic Tanny International — Alt.
14370 Eight Mile Road
Zip Code 48237
Ph. (313) 541-3100

NEW BALTIMORE
Bio-Fit System — Dual
33651 23 Mile Rd.
Zip Code 48047
Ph. (313) 725-3754

PONTIAC
Keatington Health Spa — Alt.
1755 Waldon Rd.
Zip Code 48057
Ph. (313) 391-3334

Vic Tanny International — Alt.
3432 Highland Rd.
Zip Code 48054
Ph. (313) 682-5040

Bio Fit Systems — Co-ed
2309 Airport Rd.
Zip Code 48054
Ph. (313) 666-4061

PLYMOUTH
Vic Tanny International — Dual
40700 Ann Arbor Road
Zip Code 48170
Ph. (313) 459-8890

SAGINAW
Dynamic Health Club — Alt.
5584 State St.
Zip Code 48603
Ph. (517) 792-0599

Valley Health World Inc. — Alt.
3141 Cabaret Trail
Zip Code 48603
Ph. (517) 799-5193

ST. CLAIR SHORES
Bio Fit Systems — Co-ed
24725 Harper
Zip Code 48080
Ph. (313) 771-3340

ST. JOSEPH
American Health Fitness Center
— Alt.
2848 Niles Road
Zip Code 49085
Ph. (616) 429-6711

SOUTHFIELD
Bio Fit Systems — Co-ed
26400 West 12 Mile
Zip Code 48034
Ph. (313) 356-3366

STERLING HEIGHTS
United Health Spa — Alt.
2297 18 Mile Rd.
Zip Code 48078
Ph. (313) 254-3390

TAYLOR
Bio Fit Systems — Co-ed
22805 Goodard
Zip Code 48180
Ph. (313) 287-8930

TRAVERSE CITY
Grand Traverse Health Club, Inc.
— Alt.
1129 E. Front St.
Zip Code 49684
Ph. (616) 946-2460

TROY
Total Being Fitness Center of
Troy — Women
5096 Rochester Rd.
Zip Code 48098
Ph. (313) 689-3750

Vic Tanny International — Dual
3275 Rochester Road
Zip Code 48084
Ph. (313) 689-8255

UTICA
Shape-Up Shoppe — Women
52000 Van Dyke
Zip Code 48087
Ph. (313) 739-7676

Nautilus Physical Fitness Club
— Women
45116 Cass Avenue
Zip Code 48087
Ph. (313) 739-7322

WARREN
Vic Tanny International — Alt.
38400 Dequindre
Universal City
Zip Code 48092
Ph. (313) 751-7100

Vic Tanny International — Dual
30130 Van Dyke
Zip Code 48093

WOODHAVEN
Vic Tanny International — Alt.
23303 Allen Road
Zip Code 48183
Ph. (313) 675-7400

# MINNESOTA

BLOOMINGTON
Normandale Sports & Health
Club — Dual
5250 W. 84th St.
Normandale Center
Zip Code 55437
Ph. (612) 831-2660

BROOKLYN PARK
Northaldn Park Sports & Health
Club — Dual
7624 Boone Ave., North
Zip Code 55428
Ph. (612) 425-5880

CHAMPLIN
Trim N. Sassy — Women
12359 Caville Rd.
Zip Code 55316
Ph. (612) 427-0050

DULUTH
Hal Smith's Palm Springs Health
Spa — Alt.
2215 W. Superior
Zip Code 55806
Ph. (218) 727-5039

MINNEAPOLIS
Apache Sports & Health Club —
Dual
37th & Silver Lake Rd., NE
Apache Plaza Shopping Center
Zip Code 55421
Ph. (612) 788-4066

LaSalle Sports & Health Club —
Men
LaSalle Court/Downtown
Zip Code 55402
Ph. (612) 335-6761

MINNETONKA
Fun and Fitness — Dual
12330 Wayzata Blvd., Suite 230
Zip Code 55343
Ph. (612) 546-4555

ROCHESTER
Cosmopolitan Sports & Swim
Club — Dual
1112 7th St. N.W.
Zip Code 55901
Ph. (507) 282-4445

SHOREVIEW
Trim N. Sassy — Women
1045 W. Hwy. 96
Zip Code 66112
Ph. (612) 484-3113

ST. LOUIS PARK
Park Sports & Health Club — Dual
4916 Excelsior Blvd.
Zip Code 55416
Ph. (612) 920-0212 or 927-5481

ST. PAUL
Midway Sports & Health Club —
Dual
Midway Shopping Center
Zip Code 55104
Ph. (612) 646-7491

# MISSISSIPPI

BILOXI
New Woman Figure Salon —
Women
3 Spanish Plaza, Hwy. 67
Zip Code 39532
Ph. (601) 374-2554

Kelly Lyn Figure Salon — Women
Edgewater Square
4472 Pass Rd.
Zip Code 39531
Ph. (601) 388-8511

Universal Figure Spa — Alt.
Popps Ferry Shopping Center
Zip Code 39531
Ph. (601) 388-3110

COLUMBUS
Health Club of Columbus — Alt.
2225 5th Street, North
Zip Code 39701
Ph. (601) 328-4048

GAUTIER
Kelly Lyn Figure Salon — Women
Clear Pointe Plaza
2431 Highway 90
Zip Code 39553
Ph. (601) 497-1923

HATTIESBURG
Kelly Lyn Figure Salon — Women
Lincoln Square Shopping Center
3800-B Lincoln Rd.
Zip Code 39401
Ph. (601) 545-7760

Spa Fitness Center — Alt.
4013 Hardy St.
Zip Code 39401
Ph. (601) 264-7615

JACKSON
American Fitness Center —
Women
4950 I-55 North, Jackson Plaza
Ph. (601) 981-9155

Kelly Lyn Figure Salon — Women
2535 McFadden
Apple Ridge Shopping Center
Zip Code 39204
Ph. (601) 373-0701

Kelly Lyn Figure Salon – Women
Northgate Plaza Bldg.
4436 N. State St.
Zip Code 39206
Ph. (601) 982-0156

Shotokan Karate Center & Spa –
Dual
3745 Robinson Rd.
Zip Code 39209
Ph. (601) 922-5311

Universal Fitness, Inc. – Alt.
P.O. Box 4258
Zip Code 39204
Ph. (601) 355-1535

LAUREL
Laurel Spa & Health Club Inc. –
Alt.
No. 1 North Lauren Shopping
Center
Zip Code 39440
Ph. (601) 425-4604

MERIDIAN
Kelly Lyn Figure Salon – Women
510 22nd Ave. South
Zip Code 39301
Ph. (601) 693-6066

Renaissance Fitness Centre –
Women
2131 24th Street
Zip Code 39301
Ph. (601) 483-0637

NATCHEZ
Kelly Lyn Figure Salon – Women
Trace Town Shopping Center
Zip Code 39120
Ph. (601) 442-8021

OCEAN SPRINGS
Ocean Springs Health Club &
Spa & Racquetball Club – Alt.
Highway 90 East
Zip Code 39564
Ph. (601) 875-2282

PASCAGOULA
American Health Spa – Dual
2704 Old Mobile Hwy.
Zip Code 29567
Ph. (601) 769-7217

PEARL
Universal Health Studios of Pearl
– Alt.
141 Turn-Powe Plaza
Zip Code 39208
Ph. (601) 932-1322

PICAYUNE
La Spa – Alt.
121 W. Canal St.
Zip Code 39466
Ph. (601) 798-8021

SOUTHAVEN
Dynamic Fitness Center – Alt.
1219 Stateline Road W.
Zip Code 38671
Ph. (601) 393-0926

STARKVILLE
Willie Daniel Athletic Club –
Dual
P.O. Box 656
Zip Code 39759
Ph. (601) 323-4455

TUPELO
Kelly Lyn Figure Salons –
Women
Tupelo Mall
Varsity Drive
Zip Code 38801
Ph. (601) 844-6342

New Life Health Spa – Alt.
Downtown Mall
Zip Code 38801
Ph. (601) 844-3740

WAVELAND
Kelly Lyn Figure Salon –
Women
324 U.S. Hwy. 90
Zip Code 39576
Ph. (601) 467-2905

## MISSOURI

BLUE SPRING
Blue Springs Family Fitness Cen-
ter – Alt.
1315 E. 40 Hwy.
Zip Code 64015
Ph. (816) 229-1138

CLAYTON
Vic Tanny International – Alt.
200 S. Brentwood Blvd.
Zip Code 63105
Ph. (314) 862-1900

CRESTWOOD
Vic Tanny International
9730 Watson
Zip Code 63126
Ph. (314) 822-8100

CREVE COEUR
Vic Tanny International – Alt.
12959 Olive St. Rd.
Zip Code 63141
Ph. (324) 434-2660

DELLWOOD
Vic Tanny International – Dual
9846 West Florissant
Zip Code 63136
Ph. (314) 869-6000

FLORISSANT
Vic Tanny International – Dual
225 Dunn Road
Zip Code 63031
Ph. (314) 838-2230

KANSAS CITY
KC Fitness Center – Alt.
6600 E. 87th St.
Zip Code 64138
Ph. (816) 454-2700

Mediterranean I Spa
8600 Ward Pkwy.
Zip Code 64114
Ph. (816) 333-3535

MANCHESTER
Mademoiselle Spa – Women
473 Lafayette Center
Zip Code 63011
Ph. (314) 227-5001

MARSHFIELD
Marshfield Aerobic Fitness Cen-
ter – Alt.
450 W. Jackson
Zip Code 65706
Ph. (417) 468-5210

MARYLAND HEIGHTS
Vic Tanny International – Dual
12703 Dorsett Rd.
Zip Code 63043
Ph. (314) 576-5300

MEHLVILLE
Vic Tanny International – Alt.
7425 South Lindbergh
Zip Code 63129
Ph. (314) 892-6088

ST. ANN
Vic Tanny International – Alt.
10329 St. Charles Rock Road
Zip Code 63114
Ph. (314) 423-3004

ST. CHARLES
Vic Tanny International – Alt.
I-70 at 5th Street
Mark Twain Chopping Center –
Lower Level
Zip Code 63301
Ph. (314) 723-4400

ST. JOSEPH
Magic Mirror Figure Salon –
Women
2243 N. Belt Highway
Zip Code 64506
Ph. (816) 364-5311

ST. LOUIS
Body Builders, Inc. – Dual
7090 Lansdowne
Zip Code 63109
Ph. (314) 647-1899

SPRINGFIELD
Cosmopolitan Spa
2528 S. Campbell Rd.
Old Town Shopping Center
Zip Code 65807
Ph. (417) 882-6340

Springfield Health & Fitness Center – Alt.
1536 S. Glenstone
Zip Code 65804
Ph. (417) 882-3520

## NEBRASKA

BELLEVUE
Bellevue Spa – Women
106 E. Mission
Zip Code 68005
Ph. (402) 291-5900

LINCOLN
Alpha Fitness Center – Women
140 N. 48th St.
Zip Code 68504
Ph. (402) 464-8271

OMAHA
Alpha Fitness Center – Alt.
5210 North 90th St.
Zip Code 68134
Ph. (402) 572-8502

Rockbrook Spa – Women
10820 Prairie Hills Drive
Zip Code 68144
Ph. (402) 391-7880

SCOTTSBLUFF
Nautilus Fitness Center – Dual
612 S. Beltline Hwy., East
Zip Code 69361
Ph. (308) 632-5500

SOUTH SIOUX CITY
Kim's Nautilus Fitness Center —
Dual
No. 215 S. Ridge Plaza
Zip Code 68776
Ph. 494-6433

## NEVADA

CARSON CITY
Universal Fitness Center, Inc. —
Women
1925 N. Carson St.
Zip Code 89701
Ph. (702) 883-0303

LAS VEGAS
Golden Venus Beauty & Health
Spa — Women
953-A-19 E. Sahara
Zip Code 89104
Ph. (702) 735-1223

## NEW HAMPSHIRE

CONCORD
Joy Health Spa — Women
163 Lounden Rd.
Zip Code 03301
Ph. (603) 224-5121

DERRY
Woman's World Health Spa
RFD 1 Rockingham Rd. (Rt. 28)
Zip Code 03038
Ph. (603) 434-4555

MANCHESTER
Women's World Health Spa —
Women
341 Lincoln St.
Manchester Shopping Center
Zip Code 03103
Ph. (603) 668-7580

NASHUA
Joy Health Spa — Women
Simoneau Plaza
Zip Code 03062
Ph. (603) 883-6573

PORTSMOUTH
Woman's World Health Spa —
Women
Southgate Plaza / Route 1
Zip Code 03801
Ph. (603) 431-6044 or 431-6047

SALEM
Joy Health Spa — Women
539 S. Broadway
Zip Code 03079
Ph. (603) 898-2306 or 2307

Women's World Health Spas —
Women
189 S. Broadway
Zip Code 03079
Ph. (603) 893-5716

SOUTH MERRIMACK
Woman's World Health Spa —
Women
Pennichuck Square, Route 101-A
Zip Code 03054
Ph. (603) 882-8111

## NEW JERSEY

BUENA
Buena Health & Fitness Center
Dual
Wheat Rd. & Lincoln Ave.
Zip Code 08310
Ph. (609) 697-3636

CINNAMINSON
United Health Clubs — Dual
Cinnaminson Mall
Rt. 130 & Cinnaminson Ave.
Zip Code 08077
Ph. (609) 829-6801

CLIFFSIDE PARK
Woman's World Health Spas
Women
447 Gorge Road
Zip Code 07010
Ph. (201) 941-1710

COLONIA
American Health Club — Alt.
State Hwy. No. 27
Zip Code 07067
Ph. (201) 382-6049

DEPTFORD
"Court Rooms" Spa & Racquet-
ball — Dual
1901 Deptford Center Road
Zip Code 08096
Ph. (609) 227-7000

EDISON
Edison Racquetball & Health
Club — Dual
US 1 Old Post Rd.
Zip Code 08817
Ph. (201) 287-4444

Light 'N Lovely Figure Salon —
Women
Oakwood Plaza Shopping Center
Wood Ave. & Oaktree Rd.
Zip Code 08817
Ph. (201) 548-4540

MAPLE SHADE
Bob Boone Nautilus Fitness Cen-
ters — Dual
65 Old Kings Hwy.
Zip Code 08052
Ph. (609) 234-5607

MIDLAND PARK
Woman's World Health Spa —
Women
1 Godwin Avenue
Zip Code 07432
Ph. (201) 444-5072

MORRESTOWN
New Jersey Athletic Club — Dual
451 B. Route 389
Zip Code 08057
Ph. (609) 234-4753

RAMSEY
American Women Figure Salon
Ramsey Square Shopping Center
1300 Route 17 North
Zip Code 07446
Ph. (201) 825-7707

SADDLEBROOK
American Women Figure Salon
Saddlebrook Mall
Route 46 West
Zip Code 07662
Ph. (201) 845-0386

The Health Spa at the Saddlebrook
Howard Johnson — Alt.
129 Pehle Ave.
Zip Code 07662
Ph. (201) 843-9341 or 9351, or
9441

SEA GIRT
Sea Girt Health Spa — Alt.
2100 Old Mill Plaza
Zip Code 08750
Ph. (201) 449-0790

SEWELL
Bob Boone Nautilus Fitness Cen-
ters — Dual
Route 1 P.O. Box 108-A
Zip Code 08080
Ph. (609) 589-3400

TOMS RIVER
Sands Health Spa — Dual
1861 Hooper Avenue
Zip Code 08753
Ph. (201) 255-1090

SOMERSET
Dolly's Work-Out, Inc. — Dual
1075 Easton Ave.
Zip Code 08873
Ph. (201) 846-8200

SOMERS POINT
Sands Health Spa — Alt.
New Hampshire & 7th Street
Zip Code 08753
Ph. (609) 653-8004 (11)

SUCCASUNNA
Roxbury Nautilus — Dual
Aerobic Medical Fitness Center
35 Route 10
Zip Code 07876
Ph. (201) 927-0478

VOORHEES
Club Nautilus of Echelon — Dual
15 Echelon Mall
Zip Code 08043
Ph. (609) 772-0902

WAYNE
Club Nautilus of Willowbrook —
Dual
Willowbrook Mall
Zip Code 07470
Ph. (201) 785-2110

## NEW MEXICO

CLOVIS
Executive Health Spa — Men
1321 Thorton
Zip Code 88101
Ph. (505) 762-2049

HOBBS
Golden Life Health Spa — Dual
612 N. Turner
Zip Code 88240
Ph. (505) 393-7379 or 393-9181

**ROSWELL**
Golden Life Health Spa   Dual
200 W. Hobbs
Zip Code 88201
Ph. (505) 623-4100

**SANTA FE**
Health Spa & Racquet Club
Dual
1601 St. Michaels Drive
Zip Code 87501
Ph. (505) 982-2657

**FARMINGTON**
The Athletic Club   Alt.
207 E. Main St.
Zip Code 87401
Ph. (505) 325-5454

# NEW YORK

**ALBANY**
American Health & Racquet
Club, Inc.   Dual
636 Albany Shaker Rd.
Zip Code 12211
Ph. (518) 458-7400

Nautilus Total Conditioning –
Dual
900 Central Ave.
P.O. Box 6253
Century II Mall
Zip Code 12206
Ph. (518) 458-7144

The Body Works
583 New Scotland Ave.
Zip Code 12208
Ph. (518) 489-4475

Spa Lady   Women
Wolf Road Park, Metro Drive
Zip Code 12205
Ph. (518) 459-6664 or 6665

**AMHERST**
American Health Fitness &
Racquet Center   Dual
3880 E. Robinson St.
Zip Code 14120
Ph. (716) 691-4292

**AUBURN**
New American Fitness Center
Alt.
276 Grant Avenue
Zip Code 13021
Ph. (315) 255-1932

**BROOKLYN**
Lucille Roberts Health Spa
Dual
925 Kings Hwy.
Zip Code 11223
Ph. (212) 339-0990

The Spa of Boro Park   Women
1272 53rd St.
Zip Code 11219
Ph. (212) 438-4168

**BUFFALO**
American Health Fitness Center
Dual
1208 Niagara Falls Blvd.
Zip Code 14150
Ph. (716) 837-7733

**CHEEKTOWAGA**
Sophisticated Lady Fitness
Salon – Women
1450 French Rd.
Zip Code 14043
Ph. (716) 668-6756

**CLIFTON PARK**
North Country Nautilus – Dual
Rt. 9 & 146, Clifton Park Plaza
Zip Code 12065
Ph. (518) 383-1399

**CLARENCE**
American Health Fitness Center
– Alt.
4401 Transit Road
Zip Code 14221
Ph. (716) 631-8350

Nautilus Fitness Center – Dual
4917 Transit Road
Zip Code 14221
Ph. (716) 631-9280

**DEPEW**
Nautilus Fitness Center – Dual
4721 Broadway
Zip Code 14043
Ph. (716) 681-8511

**FOREST HILLS**
Viking Health Spa – Alt.
111-20 Queens Blvd.
Zip Code 11375
Ph. (212) 520-9000

**LOCKPORT**
American Lady Figure Salon of
Lockport   Women
5885 S. Transit Rd.
Zip Code 14094
Ph. (716) 625-2211

**NEW HARTFORD**
All American Fitness Center
Dual
Kellogg Road Mall
Zip Code 13413
Ph. (315) 735-2219

**ORCHARD PARK**
American Lady Figure Salon of
Orchard Park   Women
S-3344 Southwestern Blvd.
Zip Code 14127
Ph. (716) 675-7455

**PIERMONT**
Diplomat Health Spa – Dual
Route 9W
Zip Code 10968
Ph. (914) 359-2401

**ROCHESTER**
American Health Fitness Center
– Alt.
Perinton Hills Mall
Fairport
Zip Code 14450
Ph. (716) 223-0607

American Health Fitness Center
– Dual
2345 Buffalo Road
Zip Code 14624
Ph. (716) 247-8060

American Health Fitness Center
– Dual
Ridgemont Plaza
2831 Ridge Road West Greece
Greece
Zip Code 14616
Ph. (716) 225-6600

American Health Fitness Center
– Alt.
100 Kings Rd.
Irondequoit
Zip Code 14617
Ph. (716) 266-8470

American Health Fitness Center
– Alt.
Henrietta Townline Plaza
3047 Henrietta Rd.
Zip Code 14623
Ph. (716) 424-3990

**SMITHTOWN**
Smithtown Landing Health Spa
– Alt.
620 Landing Rd.
Zip Code 11787
Ph. (516) 265-6195

**SYRACUSE**
Body Works Fitness Center –
Alt.
Geddes Shopping Center
527 Charles Ave.
Zip Code 13209
Ph. (315) 488-2831

Medical Sports Fitness Center
– Dual
Rt. 11, Ponderosa Plaza
Zip Code 13211
Ph. (315) 454-3204

**SYRACUSE (DeWITT)**
Kelly's Fitness Center – Men
3152 Erie Blvd. East
Zip Code 13214
Ph. (315) 446-3097

**TROY**
The Body Works – Dual
720 6th Avenue
Zip Code 12182
Ph. (518) 235-8485

**UTICA**
"The Club" (Nautilus at the
Sheraton) – Dual
200 Genesee Street
Zip Code 13502
Ph. (315) 735-8527

**VESTAL**
21st Century Health Spa
3108 Vestal Pkwy., East
Zip Code 13850

**VICTOR**
The Nautilus Athletic Center of
Rochester, Inc. – Co-ed
10 Railroad Street
Whistlestop Arcade
Zip Code 14564
Ph. (716) 924-7350

**WATERTOWN**
Fitness For Life Center – Dual
Globe Mall – Court St.
Zip Code 13601
Ph. (315) 788-3151

WILLIAMSVILLE
Omega Fitness Centres, Ltd. -
Dual
480 Evans Street
Zip Code 14221
Ph. (716) 634-1094

Sophisticated Lady Fitness Salon
- Women
8300 Transit Rd.
Zip Code 14221
Ph. (716) 688-0756

The Fitness Center of E. Hills
- Dual
4695 Transit Rd.
Zip Code 14221
Ph. (716) 634-4350

## NORTH CAROLINA

ASHEVILLE
Spas International, Inc.   Alt.
Turtle Creek Shopping Center
P.O. Box 15324
Zip Code 28803
Ph. (704) 274-7980

Spa Lady & Spa Fitness Center
- Alt.
Turtle Creek Shopping Center
Zip Code 28803
Ph. (704) 274-5900

Spa Lady Fitness Center
Women
Innsbruck Mall, 85 Tunnel Rd.
Zip Code 28108
Ph. (704) 258-9345

BURLINGTON
North Carolina Fitness Center -
Alt.
1805 South Church
Zip Code 27215
Ph. (919) 227-0173

CARY
Cary Spa Health Club   Dual
702 Western Boulevard Extension
Zip Code 27511
Ph. (919) 467-1001

CHAPEL HILL
Chapel Hill Spa Health Club -
Dual
Eastgate Shopping Center
Zip Code 27514
Ph. (919) 942-8714

CHARLOTTE
Cosmopolitan Spa Inc.   Alt.
727 Sharon Amity Rd.
Zip Code 28211
Ph. (704) 364-1771

Jack La Lanne   Men
5004 Albermarle Rd.
Zip Code 28212
Ph. (704) 535-7830

International Fitness Center -
Alt.
4335 Monroe Road
Zip Code 28218
Ph. (704) 372-4400

Spa Lady Fitness Center -
Women
3154 Freedom Dr.
Zip Code 28208
Ph. (704) 394-2313

Spa Lady Fitness Center
3120 Eastway Dr.
Zip Code 28205
Ph. (704) 535-2811

Spa Lady Fitness Center
5401 S. Boulevard
Zip Code 28210
Ph. (704) 525-2219

DURHAM
North Carolina Fitness Center
Women
Lakewood Shopping Center
2000 Chapel Hill Rd.
Zip Code 27707
Ph. (919) 489-6575

ELIZABETH CITY
Eternal Spring Health Spa
Southgate Mall
P.O. Box 1777
Zip Code 27909
Ph. (919) 335-0860

FAYETTEVILLE
Bordeaux Spa Fitness Center
Alt.
Boone Trail Extention
P.O. Box 64745
Zip Code 28306
Ph. (919) 483-6032

GASTONIA
Cosmopolitan Spa of Gaston Mall
Inc.   Alt.
Cox Rd. & Franklin Blvd., Gaston
Mall
Zip Code 28052
Ph. (704) 865-9588

Spa Lady Fitness Center
Women
Akers Shopping Center
Zip Code 28052
Ph. (704) 864-7758

GREENSBORO
Cosmopolitan Health Spa - Alt.
Oakcrest Shopping Center
2437 Battleground Ave.
Zip Code 27408
Ph. (919) 282-4100

North Carolina Fitness Center -
Women
2120 Lawndale Drive
Zip Code 27408
Ph. (919) 274-1616

GREENVILLE
The Spa - Dual
South Park Shopping Center
Zip Code 27834
Ph. (919) 756-7991

HICKORY
The Spa Fitness Center, Inc. -
Alt.
752 4th S.W.
Zip Code 28601
Ph. (704) 322-3026

HIGH POINT
Nautilus Sports and Fitness Cen-
ter
1133 E. Lexington Ave.
College Village Shopping Center
Zip Code 27262
Ph. (919) 889-3111

North Carolina Fitness Center -
Women
College Village Shopping Center
1121 E. Lexington St.
Zip Code 27262
Ph. (919) 883-1418

JONESVILLE
Foothills Nautilus - Dual
228 N. Bridge St.
Zip Code 28642
Ph. (919) 835-1230

KANNAPOLIS
Nautilus Fitness Center - Dual
615 N. Cannon Blvd.
Zip Code 28081
Ph. (704) 932-8000

RALEIGH
Spa Health Club - Dual
6148 Falls of Neuse Road
Zip Code 27609
Ph. (919) 876-0278

ROCKY MOUNT
Rocky Mountain Figure & Health
Spa - Women
213 Dominick Drive
Zip Code 27801
Ph. (919) 977-1767

SALISBURY
International Figure Salon -
Women
Towne Mall Shopping Center
Zip Code 28144
Ph. (704) 637-2350

Salisbury Nautilus Fitness Center - Dual
120 Mahaley Ave.
Zip Code 28144
Ph. (704) 637-3544

WINSTON-SALEM
Nautilus Elite - Dual
301 Executive Park Blvd.
Zip Code 27103
Ph. (919) 765-4651

North Carolina Fitness Center -
Women
Sherwood Plaza Shopping Center
3376 Robinhood Rd.
Zip Code 27106
Ph. (919) 765-7750

## OHIO

AKRON
Vic Tanny International - Dual
Fairlawn Plaza
Zip Code 44313
Ph. (216) 836-9121

Vic Tanny International - Dual
1220 Brittain Rd.
Zip Code 44310
Ph. (216) 633-8289

Scandinavian Spa   Alt.
Summit Mall - W. Market St.
Zip Code 44310
Ph. (216) 867-6041

Scandinavian Spa -- Alt.
1083 E. Tallmadge Ave.
Zip Code 44310
Ph. (216) 630-2200

**ASHLAND**
New Life Fitness Center – Alt.
2163 Claremont Ave.
Zip Code 44805
Ph. (419) 289-2229

**BELLEFONTAINE**
New Life Health Spa – Alt.
Hyland Hills Plaza
Zip Code 43311
Ph. (513) 593-8015

**CANTON**
Vic Tanny International – Dual
4634 Belden Village Ave. N.W.
Belden Village Shopping Center
Zip Code 44718
Ph. (216) 492-9230

Scandinavian Health Spa – Alt.
3105 Whipple Ave. N.W.
Zip Code 44708
Ph. (216) 447-3439

**CELINA**
New Life Health Spa - Alt.
107 E. Forest St.
Zip Code 45822
Ph. (419) 586-7735

**CENTERVILLE**
Moore's Nautilus Fitness Center,
Inc. – Alt.
8010 McEwen Rd.
Zip Code 45459
Ph. (513) 435-4774

**CINCINNATI**
Cincinnati Nautilus Club – Dual
11275 Chester Rd.
Zip Code 45246
Ph. (513) 772-2054

Golden Tee Health Spa – Alt.
2241 Sharon Rd.
Zip Code 45241
Ph. (513) 771-5523

Spa Lady Figure Fitness Center
– Women
441 E. Kemper Rd.
Zip Code 45246
Ph. (513) 671-0830

Spa Lady Figure Fitness Center
– Women
6490 Glenway Avenue
Zip Code 45211
Ph. (513) 574-5150

Spa Lady Figure Fitness Center
– Women
9351 Colerain Ave.
Zip Code 45239
Ph. (513) 385-7358

Vic Tanny International – Dual
9700 Colerain Ave.
Prospect Square
Colerain
Zip Code 43916
Ph. (512) 385-5523

Vic Tanny International
8040 Reading Rd.
Zip Code 45237
Ph. (513) 821-9100

Vic Tanny International
3267 Westbourne Dr.
Western Hills
Zip Code 45211
Ph. (513) 922-1731

Total Women Fitness Center –
Women
11362 Princeton Pike
Zip Code 45246
Ph. (513) 671-1500

**CLEVELAND**
Fitness & Athletic Training Cen
ter of Mill Creek Racquet Club –
Dual
18909 South Miles
Zip Code 44128
Ph. (216) 662-9001

Vic Tanny International – Alt.
Southpark Shopping Center
West 130th & Pearl Rd.
Parma Heights
Zip Code 44130
Ph. (216) 845-4161

Vic Tanny International – Alt.
Shore Center Shopping Center
22460 Shore Center Dr.
Euclid
Zip Code 44123
Ph. (216) 731-7851

Vic Tanny International – Alt.
5445 Mayfield Rd.
Lyndhurst
Zip Code 44124
Ph. (216) 449-4855

Vic Tanny International – Alt.
19707 Center Ridge Rd.
Rocky River
Zip Code 44111
Ph. (216) 331-7070

Vic Tanny International – Dual
14783 Pearl Rd.
Strongsville
Zip Code 44138
Ph. (216) 238-1616

Vic Tanny International – Dual
8000-21 Plaza Blvd.
Mentor
Zip Code 44060
Ph. (216) 255-3003

**COLUMBUS**
Scandinavian Health Spa – Dual
4290 Macsway
Zip Code 43227
Ph. (614) 863-1163

Scandinavian Health Spa – Dual
1987 Morse Road
Zip Code 43229

Spa Lady – Women
3427 South Blvd.
Zip Code 43204
Ph. (614) 279-9562

The Spa at Dublin – Women
6520 Riverside Dr.
Zip Code 43017
Ph. (614) 764-0126

Spa Lady Figure Fitness Center –
Women
3763 S. High St.
Great Southern Shopping Center
Zip Code 43207
Ph. (614) 491-3570

Spa Lady Figure Fitness Center –
Women
5949 E. Main St., Carnaby Mall
Zip Code 43227
Ph. (614) 866-9181

Spa Lady Figure Fitness Center –
Women
5992 Westerville Rd.
Zip Code 43081
Ph. (614) 890-2621

Spa Lady Figure Fitness Center –
Women
1222 Kenny Rd.
Kenny Centre Mall
Zip Code 43211
Ph. (614) 459-3131

**DAYTON**
Holiday Health Spa – Alt.
1020 West Centerville Road
Zip Code 45459
Ph. (513) 434-8738

Holiday Health Spa – Alt.
3535 Salem Avenue
Zip Code 45406
Ph. (513) 277-8971

Holiday Health Spa – Alt.
3022 Wilmington Avenue
Zip Code 45429
Ph. (513) 294-1418

John Powell Sports Center, Inc.
– Dual
5623 Old Troy Pike
Zip Code 45424
Ph. (513) 233-9337

The Rike's Spa – Women
2nd and Main St.
Zip Code 45402
Ph. (513) 225-8024

The Total Woman Health Club –
Women
South Town Center
2058 Miamisburg-Centerville Blvd.
Zip Code 45459
Ph. (513) 435-6100

Vic Tanny Vita-Life Health Salon
– Alt.
3180 Kettering Blvd.
Zip Code 45439
Ph. (513) 298-0281

Vic Tanny Vita-Life Health Salon
– Alt.
3453 Sibenthaler Ave.
Zip Code 45406
Ph. (513) 276-2118

**DEFIANCE**
Vita-Life Health Spa – Alt.
1846 East 2nd Street
Zip Code 43512
Ph. (419) 782-8223

**ELYRIA**
Scandinavian Health Spa – Dual
41162 Giswald Rd.
Zip Code 44035
Ph. (216) 777-6499

**ENGLEWOOD**
Holiday Health Spa – Alt.
20 W. Wenger Road
Zip Code 45322
Ph. (513) 836-9616

Moore's Nautilus – Alt.
606 Taywood Rd.
Zip Code 45322
Ph. (513) 836-2654

**FAIRBORN**
Holiday Health Spa – Alt.
1222 Kauffman Avenue
Zip Code 45324
Ph. (513) 879-2881

**FAIRFIELD**
Olympian Fitness World, Inc.
Men
32 Donald Drive
Zip Code 45014
Ph. (513) 896-9030

**FINDLAY**
Findlay Circuit COurts    Dual
1219 W. Main Cross
Zip Code 45840
Ph. (419) 424-1970

New Life Health Spa    Alt.
1645 Tiffin Ave.
Zip Code 45840
Ph. (419) 424-9551

**HOLLAND**
Family Nautilus Fitness Centers
Dual
6834 Spring Valley Dr.
Zip Code 43528
Ph. (419) 866-6977

**GALION**
Slender Magic Health Center –
Alt.
11 Public Square
Zip Code 44833
Ph. (419) 468-5987

**GREENVILLE**
New Life Fitness Center – Alt.
7551 Celina Road
Zip Code 45331
Ph. (513) 548-2422

**KENTON**
Aerobics Fitness Center – Women
213 W. Columbus St.
Zip Code 43326
Ph. (419) 674-4727

**LIMA**
New Life Health Spa – Alt.
3200 Harding Highway
Easthate Plaza
Zip Code 45804
Ph. (419) 227-6800

New Life Health Spa    Dual
3101 West Elm St.
Zip Code 45805
Ph. (419) 991-8015

**MAYFIELD HEIGHTS**
**(CLEVELAND)**
Scandinavian Health Spa
Golden Gate Shopping Center
6420 Mayfield Rd.
Zip Code 44124
Ph. (216) 461-2735

**MANSFIELD**
New Life Health Spa    Alt.
1411 Lexington Ave.
Zip Code 44902
Ph. (419) 756-7152

**MARION**
New Life Health Spa    Alt.
150 Barks Rd. East
Zip Code 43302
Ph. (614) 389-4602

**MAUMEE**
21st Century Health Spa    Alt.
2584 Anthony Wayne Trail
Parkway Plaza Shopping Center
Zip Code 43537
Ph. (419) 893-9428

**MIDDLEBURG HEIGHTS**
Fitness World of Ohio Inc. –
Women
13383 Smith Rd.
Zip Codd 44130
Ph. (216) 888-5522

**NORTH OLMSTEAD**
Scandinavian Health Spa – Dual
27336 Lorain Rd.
Zip Code 44070
Ph. (216) 734-4744

**NORTH RANDALL**
**(CLEVELAND)**
Scandinavian Health Spa – Alt.
4562 Warrensville Center Road
Zip Code 44128
Ph. (216)  587-2843

**PARMA (CLEVELAND)**
Scandinavian Health Spa - Dual
6875 Ridoe Rd.
Zip Code 44129
Ph. (216) 888-8890

**PERRYSBURG**
Family Nautilus Fitness Center –
Dual
27511 Holiday Lane
Zip Code 43551
Ph. (419) 874-8769

Nautilus Country Charm, Inc. –
Dual
134 W.S. Boundary
Zip Code 43551
Ph. (419) 874-3707

**SANDUSKY**
Vic Tanny International – Alt.
Perkins Plaza
Zip Code 44870
Ph. (419) 625-0450

**SIDNEY**
New Life Health Spa – Alt.
1555 W. Michigan St.
Zip Code 45365
Ph. (513) 492-6145

**SPRINGFIELD**
Universal Health Spa — Alt.
4841 Urbana
Zip Code 45503
Ph. (513) 399-9810

**STRUTHERS**
World of Tanglewood Health
Resort – Alt.
777 Youngstown Poland Rd.
Zip Code 44471
Ph. (216) 755-9808

**TOLEDO**
Vic Tanny International – Alt.
Miracle Mile Shopping Center
4925 Jackman Rd.
Zip Code 43613
Ph. (419) 474-5708

Vic Tanny International – Dual
1123-25 N. Reynolds Rd.
Zip Code 43615
Ph. (419) 531-5148

Vic Tanny International – Dual
5215 S. Monroe Street
Sylvania
Zip Code 43623
Ph. (419) 885-4627

21st Century Health Spa – Alt.
6226 Summit St.
Merchand Landing Shopping Ctr.
Zip Code 43611
Ph. (419) 729-3941

21st Century Health Spa – Alt.
2612 Woodville Rd.
Great Eastern Shopping Center
Zip Code 43619
Ph. (419) 693-0473

21st Century Health Spa – Alt.
5115 Monroe St.
Zip Code 43623
Ph. (419) 882-0568

**TROY**
New Life Health Spa – Alt.
32 S. Weston Rd.
Zip Code 45373
Ph. (513) 339-0577

**UNIVERSITY HEIGHTS**
Fitness World – Women
2170 Warrensville Center Rd.
Zip Code 44118
Ph. (216) 371-3211

**WADSWORTH**
Willmark Fitness Center, Inc. –
Alt.
130 S. Lyman St.
Zip Code 44281
Ph. (216) 336-4824

**WAPAKONETA**
New Life Health Spa – Alt.
1201 Defiance St.
Zip Code 45895
Ph. (419) 738-9245

**WILLOWICK (CLEVELAND)**
Scandinavian Health Spa – Dual
30600 Lakeshore Blvd.
Zip Code 44094
Ph. (216) 994-9806

**WOOSTER**
New Life Fitness Center – Alt.
3400 Old Airport Rd.
Zip Code 44691
Ph. (216) 263-0444

**XENIA**
Elegant Lady – Women
55 S. Allison
Zip Code 45385
Ph. (513) 376-4322

The King's Nautilus – Men
45 S. Allison Ave.
Zip Code 45385
Ph. (513) 376-4311

## OKLAHOMA

**ALTUS**
Magic Mirror Figure Salon
Women
3004 N. Main St.
Zip Code 73521
Ph. (405) 482-5678

**ARDMORE**
Magic Mirror Figure Salon
Women
38 Tiffany Plaza
Zip Code 73401
Ph. (405) 226-2080

**BARTLESVILLE**
Nomi's Fitness Centre, Inc.   Alt.
"The Quarters" 4100 Adams Rd.
Zip Code 74003
Ph. (918) 333-4257

**DEL CITY**
Magic Mirror Figure Salon –
Women
5526 S.E. 15th St.
Zip Code 73115
Ph. (405) 670-3689

**DUNCAN**
Magic Mirror Figure Salon –
Women
4021 Highway 81 North
Zip Code 73533
Ph. (405) 252-0496

**EDMOND**
Magic Mirror Figure Salon –
Women
3413 S. Wynn Dr.
Zip Code 73034
Ph. (405) 341-7222

Nautilus Fitness Center – Alt.
514 S. Bryant
Zip Code 73034
Ph. (405) 348-3714

**ENID**
Magic Mirror Figure Salon –
Women
1010 W. Cherry St.
North Van Buren Shopping Ctr.
Zip Code 73701
Ph. (405) 237-8552

Nautilus Fitness Center – Dual
302 N. Independence
Zip Code 73701
Ph. (405) 237-1260

Moni's Fitness Centre – Alt.
2411 Heritage Trail
Zip Code 73701
Ph. (405) 242-0303

**LAWTON**
Magic Mirror Figure Salon
Women
1025 North 38th St.
Zip Code 73505
Ph. (405) 355-3413

**MOORE**
Magic Mirror Figure Salon –
Women
Peppertree Shopping Center
1336 N. Santa Fe
Zip Code 73160
Ph. (405) 799-3389

**NORMAN**
Win's Fitness World – Dual
1317 East Lindsey
Zip Code 73071
Ph. (405) 329-8514

**OKLAHOMA CITY**
Magic Mirror Figure Salon –
Women
Village Park Shopping Center
10505 North May Ave.
Zip Code 73120
Ph. (405) 751-2604

Magic Mirror Figure Salon –
Women
Reding Shopping Center
4125 S. Western
Zip Code 73109
Ph. (405) 631-6677

Magic Mirror Figure Salon –
Women
Brookhaven Shopping Center
7737 N.W. 94th St.
Zip Code 73132
Ph. (405) 721-1111

Spa Lady – Women
9230 N. Pennsylvania Ave.
Zip Code 73120
Ph. (405) 840-3381

Win's Fitness World – Dual
3013 NW 63rd
Zip Code 73112
Ph. (405) 840-3573

**PONCA CITY**
Magic Mirror Figure Salon –
Women
712 E. Prospect
Zip Code 74601
Ph. (405) 762-9027

Nomi's Fitness Center, Inc. –
Alt.
2709 No. Fourteenth
Zip Code 74601
Ph. (405) 762-5609

**SHAWNEE**
Magic Mirror Figure Salon –
Women
1615 N. Harrison St.
Zip Code 74801
Ph. (405) 275-3755

**STILLWATER**
Magic Mirror Figure Salon –
Women
712 S. Devon
Zip Code 74074
Ph. (405) 624-1854

Nautilus Fitness Center – Alt.
1515 Boomer Road
Zip Code 74074
Ph. (405) 377-9435

**TULSA**
Century Health Spa – Dual
2198-A S. Sheridan
Zip Code 74129
Ph. (918) 836-3561

Cosmopolitan Lady – Women
7875 East 51st
Fontana Shopping Center
Zip Code 74145
Ph. (918) 663-3091

**YUKON**
Magic Mirror Figure Salon –
Women
1107 Cornwell Ave.
Zip Code 73099
Ph. (405) 354-4891

## OREGON

**BEAVERTON**
Spa Figure & Fitness Center –
Women
12785 SW Jenkins Rd.
Zip Code 97005
Ph. (503) 646-4044

**BEND**
Bend Figure Salon – Women
929 NW Wall
Zip Code 97701
Ph. (503) 382-7447

**CLACKAMAS**
Fitness Unlimited – Alt.
P.O. Box 201
16200 S.E. 83nd Dr., Suite D
Zip Code 97015
Ph. (503) 655-5334

**COOS BAY**
Coos Bay Health Spa – Women
862 S. Broadway
Zip Code 97420
Ph. (503) 269-9011

**EUGENE**
Eugene Health & Fitness Center
– Alt.
2868 Williamette St.
Zip Code 97405
Ph. (503) 344-6681

Oakway Spa – Alt.
16 Oakway Mall
Zip Code 97402
Ph. (503) 343-3314

**GRESHAM**
The Gresham Athletic Club –
Dual
N.W. 1st & Miller
P.O. Box 261
Zip Code 97030
Ph. (503) 665-2126

**MEDFORD**
Palm Springs Health Spa – Alt.
313 E. 8th
Zip Code 97501
Ph. (503) 773-9014

**MILWAUKIE**
Spa Figure & Fitness Center –
Women
16037 S.E. McLoughlin Ave.
Zip Code 97222
Ph. (503) 659-9064

**PORTLAND**
Spa Figure & Fitness Center –
Alt
1936 NE 122nd Ave.
Zip Code 97230
Ph. (503) 255-4868

Spa Figure & Fitness Center –
Women
2300 SE 182nd Ave.
Zip Code 97233
Ph. (503) 665-3178

Spa Figure & Fitness Center –
Women
2714 NE Broadway
Zip Code 97232
Ph. (503) 288-7221

**SALEM**
Palm Springs Health Spa – Alt.
447 Court St., NE
Zip Code 97301
Ph. (503) 585-5502

**TIGARD**
Spa Figure & Fitness Center –
Women
11535 S.W. Pacific Hwy.
Zip Code 97223
Ph. (503) 245-1144

# PENNSYLVANIA

**ALLENTOWN**
Slim-Time Spa – Women
Parkway Shopping Center
Zip Code 18103
Ph. (215) 791-3544

The Body Factory Fitness Center
– Dual
Routes 22 & 309 at Vantage Point
Zip Code 18109
Ph. (215) 395-0590

**ARDMORE**
Nautilus of America – Co-ed
Five East Lancaster Ave.
Zip Code 19003
Ph. (215) 649-5700

**BEAVER**
Genesis Health Clubs – Alt.
575 Turnpike St.
Zip Code 15009
Ph. (412) 728-3262

**BENSALEM**
Bucks County Exercise & Athletic
Club – Dual
2746 Mechanicsville Rd.
Zip Code 19020
Ph. (215) 245-1585

**BETHLEHEM**
Slim-Time Spa – Women
Lehigh Shopping Center
Zip Code 18018
Ph. (215) 691-6212

**BLOOMSBURG**
New You Spa & Fitness Center
1123 Old Berwick Rd.
Zip Code 17815
Ph. (717) 387-0300

**BRIDGEVILLE**
Nautilus Fitness Center – Dual
419 Station St.
Zip Code 15017
Ph. (412) 257-0730

**CAMP HILL**
Mini Vacation Spa – Women
905 Kranzel Dr.
Zip Code 17011
Ph. (717) 763-4418

**CHADDS FORD**
Kirkwood Fitness Club – Dual
Route 202 & Pyle Road
RD No. 2 Box 302A
Zip Code 19317
Ph. (215) 459-5150

**CONSHOHOCKEN**
Olympic Nautilus Health Club
Plymouth Square Shopping
Center
Ridge and Butler Pikes
Zip Code 19428
Ph. (215) 828-8202

**DICKSON CITY**
Spa Fitness Centers – Alt.
Rt. 6 Scranton/Carbondale Hwy.
Zip Code 18519
Ph. (717) 346-0754

**DUBOIS**
The Olympian Fitness Center –
Dual
17 N. Main
Zip Code 15801
Ph. (814) 375-0653

**DUNCANSVILLE**
Body Boutique Spa – Women
764 Plaza
Zip Code 16635
Ph. (814) 695-4433

**ERIE**
Body Works – Women
1210 W. 26th Street
Zip Code 16508
Ph. (814) 456-5334

Universal Spa Lady – Women
Millcreek Mall No. 647
Zip Code 16510
Ph. (814) 686-5461

**EXTON**
Spa Health & Fitness Center –
Alt.
102 Exton Square Mall
Zip Code 19341
Ph. (215) 363-1176

**GETTYSBURG**
Mini Vacation Spa – Women
RD 8, Box 256
Zip Code 17325
Ph. (717) 334-0072

**HANOVER**
Slim Time Beauty Spa of Hanover
– Women
Clearview Shopping Center
Zip Code 17331
Ph. (717) 632-8011

**HARRISBURG**
Bently Club – Dual
2301 Grimes Dr.
Zip Code 17112
Ph. (717) 545-4231

Slim Time Beauty Spa of Harris-
burg – Women
East Mall (Annex)
Zip Code 17111
Ph. (717) 564-5544

**JENKINTOWN**
Club Nautilus of Abington, Inc. –
Dual
817 Old York Road
Zip Code 19046
Ph. (215) 576-0303

**KING OF PRUSSIA**
Body Technics, Nautilus Fitness
Center – Dual
150 Allendale Road
Zip Code 19406
Ph. (215) 265-9001

United Health Clubs, Inc. – Alt.
150 W. DeKalb Pike
Zip Code 19406
Ph. (215) 337-1661

**LANCASTER**
The Lancaster Health Spa I
Alt.
1107 Park City Center
Zip Code 17601
Ph. (717) 299-3631

The Lancaster Health Spa – Alt.
East Towne Mall
Zip Code 17604
Ph. (717) 291-5959

**LANGHORNE**
American Health Fitness Center –
Dual
130 Middletown Blvd.
Zip Code 19040
Ph. (215) 752-9506

Club Nautilus – Dual
2300 E. Lincoln Hwy.
Zip Code 19047
Ph. (215) 752-7676

**LEBANON**
New Figure Spa – Women
1604 E. Cumberland St.
Zip Code 17042
Ph. (717) 274-3439

**MECHANICSBURG**
Body Boutique Spa – Women
5600 Carlisle Pike
Zip Code 17055
Ph. (717) 697-0387

**MONROEVILLE (PITTSBURGH)**
Spa Lady – Women
4089 William Penn Hwy.
Zip Code 15146
Ph. (412) 856-7850

**MOOSIC**
The Lancaster Health Spa II
Alt.
U.S. Rt. 11 Birney Plaza
Zip Code 19507
Ph. (717) 961-1160

**PAOLI**
Nautilus of Paoli – Dual
1 Spring St.
Zip Code 19301
Ph. (215) 296-0433

PHILADELPHIA
American Health Fitness Center
9185 Roosevelt Blvd.
Zip Code 19114
Ph. (215) 676-9110

Club Nautilus of Center City
Dual

Rittenhouse Regency
229 S. 18th St.
Zip Code 19103
Ph. (215) 546-1218

Norco Health Spa — Dual
Krewston Rd. & Grant Ave.
Zip Code 19115
Ph. (215) 671-9969

Philadelphia Aerobic & Nautilus
Fitness Center — Dual
2901 W. Cheltenham Ave.
Zip Code 19150
Ph. (215) 885-0540

Philadelphia Aquatic & Exercise
Center — Dual
3600 Grant Ave.
Zip Code 19114
Ph. (215) OR7-0400

The Bourse Nautilus — Dual
21 S. 5th Street
Zip Code 19106
Ph. (215) 627-3545

United Health Clubs — Alt.
4600 City Line Ave.
Zip Code 19131
Ph. (215) 879-5050

PITTSBURGH
Body Technics — Dual
3609 Forbes Ave.
Zip Code 15213
Ph. (412) 683-0900

Nautilus Fitness Center — Dual
5850 Ellsworth Ave.
Zip Code 15232
Ph. (412) 363-0505

PLEASANT HILLS
(PITTSBURGH)
Spa Lady — Women
Rt. 51
Southland Shopping Center
Zip Code 15236
Ph. (412) 655-9190

READING
fitness World Nautilus Spa — Dual
134 N. 5th St.
Zip Code 19603
Ph. (215) 378-5000

Mini-Vacation Spa — Women
Antietam Valley Shopping Center
Zip Code 19606
Ph. (215) 779-2427

Woman's World Mini Spa's Inc. —
Women
5th St. Highway
Nichols Shopping Center
Zip Code 19605
Ph. (215) 921-3111

SHAMOKIN
New You Spa & Fitness Center -
Alt.
Rt. 61, Anthra Plaza
Zip Code 17872
Ph. (717) 648-6801

SPRINGFIELD
Spa Health & Fitness Centers —
Alt.
Springfield Shopping Center
147 State Rd.
Zip Code 19064
Ph. (215) 328-9430

SPRINGHOUSE
Spa Health & Fitness Centers —
Alt.
Village Shopping Center (Lower
Level)
Zip Code 19477
Ph. (215) 646-2700

STATE COLLEGE
Nautilus Human Performance
Center — Dual
134 E. Foster Ave.
Zip Code 16801
Ph. (814) 238-2038

Nittany Nautilus — Dual
131 S. Pugh Street
Zip Code 16801
Ph. (814) 234-4225

UNIONTOWN
Fun and Fitness Health Spa —
Women
29 W. Main
Zip Code 15401
Ph. (412) 439-4501

Uniontown Spa & Fitness Center
— Men
29 W. Main
Zip Code 15401
Ph. (412) 439-1920

WASHINGTON
Terrace Trim — Women
326 Terrace Avenue
Zip Code 15301
Ph. (412) 228-8410

WEST CHESTER
Spa Health & Fitness Centers —
Alt.
1103 Westchester Pike
Zip Code 19380
Ph. (215) 431-7000

WILKES-BARRE
Spa Petite — Women
1145 Highway 315
Zip Code 18702
Ph. (717) 825-8549

WILLIAMSPORT
The Oasis Health Spa — Women
2310 Lycoming Creek Rd.
Zip Code 17701
Ph. (717) 322-6389

The Rose Garden Health Spa -
Women
921 Westminster Dr.
Zip Code 17701
Ph. (717) 322-4641

WOODLYN
The Sports Factory, Inc. — Dual
Woodlyn Square Center
Macdale Blvd. & Fairview Rd.
Zip Code 19094
Ph. (215) 833-2000

YORK
Slim-Times Spas — Women
North Mall
Zip Code 17404
Ph. (717) 767-6532

## RHODE ISLAND

BRISTOL
Woman's World Health Spa -
Women
Bristol Shopping Center
20 Gooding Avenue
Zip Code 02809
Ph. (401) 253-2020

CRANSTON
Woman's World Health Spa —
Women
905 Pontiac Avenue
Zip Code 02360
Ph. (401) 467-7750

LINCOLN
Woman's World Health Spa —
Women
Route 115 — Lincoln Mall
Zip Code 02865
Ph. (401) 333-2024

NORTH KINGSTON
American Health Fitness Center
of N. Kingston — Dual
7540 Post Road
Zip Code 02852
Ph. (401) 295-9711

NORTH PROVIDENCE
American Women Fitness Center
1920 Mineral Spring Ave.
Zip Code 02904
Ph. (401) 353-9230

Women's World Health Spa
Women
1420 Mineral Spring Ave.
Zip Code 02904
Py. (401) 353-5510

PAWTUCKET
Woman's World Health Spa -
Women
727 East Avenue
Zip Code 02860
Ph. (401) 722-3054

PROVIDENCE
American Health Fitness Center
— Dual
Garden City Shopping Center
170 Hillside Ave.
Cranston
Zip Code 02920
Ph. (401) 944-7353

SMITHFIELD
The Total Women Figure Salon
Village Plaza
375 Putnam Pike Store No. 7
Zip Code 02917
Ph. (401) 231-9330

WARWICK
American Health Fitness Center
— Alt.
475 Warwick Mall
Zip Code 02886
Ph. (401) 738-1250

American Women Fitness Center
— Women
2462 Warwick Avenue
Zip Code 02886
Ph. (401) 739-8020

WOONSOCKET
Woman's World Health Spa —
Women
390 Clinton St.
Zip Code 02895
Ph. (401) 762-1465

## SOUTH CAROLINA

ANDERSON
Spa South of Carolina — Alt.
3420 N. Main Street
Market Place Shopping Center
Zip Code 20624
Ph. (803) 224-7934

Spa Lady Fitness Center —
Women
205 S. 28 By-Pass
Southgate Shopping Center
Zip Code 29621
Ph. (803) 224-7431

CAMDEN
Camden Fitness Center, Inc. —
Alt.
1031 Broad Street
Sip Code 29020
Ph. (803) 432-0596

CHARLESTON
International Fitness Center —
Dual
5900 Rivers Ave.
Zip Code 29405
Ph. (803) 554-6895

Lady International Fitness Center
— Women
1650 Sam Rittenburg Blvd.
Zip Code 29407
Ph. (803) 556-0620

COLUMBIA
Holidah Health & Fitness Center
1597 Broad River Road
Zip Code 29210

Holiday Health & Fitness Center
2204 Beltline Blvd.
North Richland Mall
Zip Code 29204

Spa Lady — Women
2768 Decker Blvd.
Zip Code 29206
Ph. (803) 788-1150

Spa Lady — Women
3315 Broad River Rd.
Widewater Square
Zip Code 29210
Ph. (803) 798-7344

Spa Lady — Women
6740 Garners Ferry Rd.
Zip Code 29209
Ph. (803) 776-3411

FLORENCE
Continental Spa — Women
1641 W. Palmetto St.
Zip Code 29501
Ph. (803) 662-4552

International Fitness Center —
Alt.
1930 W. Palmetto St.
Zip Code 29501
Ph. (803) 665-5780

Olympia Health Spa
608 W. Evans
Zip Code 29501
Ph. (803) 669-4610

GREENVILLE
Holiday Health & Fitness Center
630 S. Pleasantburg Drive
Zip Code 29607

Spa South of Greenville — Alt.
P.O. Box 5551
385 at Roper Mt.
Zip Code 29607
Ph. (803) 288-8774

Spa Lady Fitness Center —
Women
Wade Hampton Mall
Wade Hampton Blvd.
Zip Code 29609
Ph. (803) 233-1625

Today's Women of Greenville —
Women
730 Cedar Lane Plaza
Zip Code 29611
Ph. (803) 246-4730

LEXINGTON
Spa Lady Fitness Center —
Women
Hwy. 378
Village Square Shopping Center
Zip Code 29072
Ph. (803) 359-5185

MT. PLEASANT
Lady International — Women
Fairmont Shopping Center
1035 N. Highway 17 By-Pass
Zip Code 29464
Ph. (803) 881-1178

NORTH AUGUSTA
Spa Lady Fitness Center —
Women
A-3 East Martin Town Rd.
North Augusta Plaza
Zip Code 29841
Ph. (803) 278-1150

ORANGEBURG
Orangeburg Health & Fitness
Center — Alt.
5534 Russell St. N.E.
Sip Code 29115
Ph. (803) 536-0000

ROCK HILL
Rock Hill World of Fitness — Alt.
358 Park Avenue
Zip Code 29730
Ph. (803) 324-5291

Spa Lady Fitness Center —
Women
Beatty Shopping Center
Cherry Road
Zip Code 29730
Ph. (803) 324-4030

SPARTANBURG
Regency Health Spa — Alt.
K-Mart Shopping Center
800 Garner Rd.
Zip Code 29301
Ph. (803) 585-8339

Spa Lady Fitness Center —
Women
2015 N.Church Place
Zip Code 29303
Ph. (803) 585-7162

Spa Lady Fitness Center —
Women
Fernwood Glendale Dr.
Zip Code 29302
Ph. (803) 585-1654

SUMMERVILLE
International Fitness Center —
Alt.
1185 Dorchester Rd.
Dorchester Village Mall
Zip Code 29483
Ph. (803) 875-1130

SUMTER
International Fitness Center —
Dual
443 Broad St.
Zip Code 29150
Ph. (803) 775-7379

WEST COLUMBIA
Spa Lady — Women
1472 Charleston Hwy.
West End Square
Zip Code 29169
Ph. (803) 791-5424

## SOUTH DAKOTA

RAPID CITY
Spa '80 for Women — Women
508 6th St.
Zip Code 57701
Ph. (605) 342-8080

SIOUX FALLS
International Health Spa — Alt.
3021 East 10th St.
Zip Code 57103
Ph. (605) 334-1440

## TENNESSEE

ALCOA
Nationwide Fitness Center & Spa
— Dual
Midland Shopping Center
Zip Code 37701
Ph. (615) 984-7844

ANTIOCH
Kelly Lyn Figure Salons —
Women
Hickory Hollow Court Yard
867 Bell Rd.
Zip Code 37013
Ph. (615) 834-6776

ATHENS
Nationwide Health Spa — Alt.
214 North White St.
Zip Code 37303
Ph. (615) 745-3326

BRISTOL
Kelly Lyn Figure Salons –
Women
Southgate Shopping Center
Voluntter Pkwy.
Zip Code 37620
Ph. (615) 968-7322

CHATTANOOGA
Fitness World – Women
4779 Brainerd Rd.
Zip Code 37411
Ph. (615) 894-7545

Kelly Lyn Figure Salons –
Women
Ridgewood Village Shopping
Center
5611 Ringgold Rd.
Zip Code 37412
Ph. (615) 894-7446

Slimette/Chattanooga Health Spa
Dual
4200 N. Access Rd.
Zip Code 37415
Ph. (615) 877-2411 or 877-6883

21st Century Health Spa – Alt.
5647 Brainerd Rd.
Zip Code 37411
Ph. (615) 894-0022

21st Century Health Spa – Alt.
364 Northgate Mall
Zip Code 37415
Ph. (615) 877-3559

CLARKSVILLE
Kelly Lyn Figure Salons –
Women
Tradewinds North S.C.
Ft. Campbell Highway
Zip Code 37040
Ph. (615) 552-3401

Sum Figure of Clarksville –
Women
30 Crossland Ave.
Zip Code 37040
Ph. (615) 552-4308

Universal Health & Fitness
Centers – Dual
1990 Madison St.
Zip Code 37040
Ph. (615) 552-3415

CLEVELAND
Holiday Spa – Alt.
903 Keith St., N.W.
Zip Code 37311
Ph. (615) 479-4551

Woman's World of Health, Inc.
702 17th Street, NW, Suite C
Zip Code 37311
Ph. (615) 479-8534

COLUMBIA
Spartan Health Spa, Inc. – Alt.
1211 Hatcher Lane
Zip Code 38401
Ph. (615) 381-9097

COOKEVILLE
Centurion Fitness Centre, Inc. –
Alt.
135 N. Washington Ave.
Zip Code 38501
Ph. (615) 528-6595

The Body Shoppe – Women
221 East Eighth
Zip Code 38501
Ph. (615) 526-3214

CROSSVILLE
Centurion Fitness Center – Alt.
110 Hayes Street
Zip Code 38555
Ph. (615) 484-2517

Nautilus Fitness & Racquetball
Center – Dual
Woodmere Mall
Zip Code 38555
Ph. (615) 484-9644

DAYTON
Rhea County Health Club – Alt.
Richland Park Shopping Center
Zip Code 37321
Ph. (615) 775-5222

DUNLOP
Valley Health Spa, Inc. – Dual
P.O. Box 125 – Hwy. 127
Zip Code 37327
Ph. (615) 949-4207

FRANKLIN
Kelly Lyn Figure Salons –
Women
Heritage Square, Hillsboro Rd.
Zip Code 37064
Ph. (615) 790-7583

GALLATIN
Gallatin Health Spa – Alt.
270 E. Main St.
Zip Code 37066
Ph. (615) 452-0054

JACKSON
Kelly Lyn Figure Salon – Women
24 Federal Drive, Suite 242
Zip Code 38301
Ph. (901) 668-7500

JOHNSON CITY
Cosmopolitan Spa Int. – Alt.
2011 North Roan
Zip Code 37601
Ph. (615) 282-0771

Kelly Lyn Figure Salon No. 12 –
Women
1313 Indian Ridge Rd.
Zip Code 37601
Ph. (615) 928-6485

KINGSPORT
Cosmopolitan Spa of Kingsport –
Alt.
Kings Giant Plaza
Zip Code 37660
Ph. (615) 246-8611

Kelly Lyn – Figure Salon No. 13
– Women
1401 E. Stone Dr.
Zip Code 37660
Ph. (615) 247-6185

KNOXVILLE
Kelly Lyn Figure Salons –
Women
7209 Chapman Hwy.
Zip Code 37920
Ph. (615) 573-8946

Kelly Lyn Figure Salons –
Women
Halls Plaza
7118½ Maynardsville Hwy.
Zip Code 37918
Ph. (615) 922-7727

Paschal International Spa – Men
137 Western Plaza
Zip Code 37919
Ph. (615) 693-9323

Vic Tanny Health & Racquet
Club – Men & Women
1501 Kirby Road
Zip Code 37919
Ph. (615) 588-6461

McMINNVILLE
Odyssey Spa – Alt.
Route 3
Box 470-B
Zip Code 37110
Ph. (615) 668-9553

MADISON
Kelly Lyn Figure Salon No. 2 –
Women
1994 Gallatin Rd. North
Zip Code 37115
Ph. (615) 859-4105

World Class Gym, Inc. – Men
135 Gallatin Road
Zip Code 37115
Ph. (615) 868-2838

MARYVILLE
Kelly Lyn Figure Salon –
Women
1622 W. Broadway
Cornerstone Square
Zip Code 37801
Ph. (615) 982-3501

MEMPHIS
Fitness World – Women
3024 Covington Pike
Zip Code 38128
Ph. (901) 388-3220

French Riviera Spa – Alt.
4029 Hawkins Mill Rd.
Zip Code 38128
Ph. (901) 382-2960

Fitness World – Women
2725 S. Mendenhall
Zip Code 38118
Ph. (901) 362-9441

Kelly Lyn Figure Salon No. 44 –
Women
845 S. White Station Rd.
Zip Code 38117
Ph. (901) 682-6636

Kelly Lyn Figure Salon No. 5 –
Women
2850 Austin Peay – Suite 134
Zip Code 38128
Ph. (901) 372-4550

Kelly Lyn Figure Salon No. 6 –
Women
1239 Winchester
Zip Code 38116
Ph. (901) 332-2685

Nautilus Training Center of
Memphis – Dual
853 S. White Station
Zip Code 38117
Ph. (901) 761-2211 or 761-2210

The French Riviera Spa – Alt . . .
The French Riviera Spa – Alt.
4075 Summer Avenue
Zip Code 38122
Ph. (901) 323-5519

The French Riviera Health Club –
Alt.
4641 American Way
Zip Code 38118
Ph. (901) 365-4180

**MORRISTOWN**
Health World International Spa –
Alt.
Downtown Shopping Mall
Zip Code 37814
Ph. (615) 581-3802

**MURFREESBORO**
Kelly Lyn Figure Salon –
Women
1250 Northwest Broad St.
The Mall
Zip Code 37130
Ph. (615) 895-2380

Southeastern Health Spa, Inc. –
Alt.
Jackson Heights Plaza
Zip Code 37130
Ph. (615) 895-0604

**NASHVILLE**
Cosmopolitan Spa International,
Inc. – Alt.
3820 Cleghorn Ave.
Zip Code 37215
Ph. (615) 383-5802

Cosmopolitan Spa International,
Inc. – Alt.
707 Two Mile Pike
Goodlettsville
Zip Code 37072
Ph. (615) 859-3845

Cosmopolitan Spa International,
Inc. – Alt.
Fairlane Shopping Center
4994 Nolensville Rd.
Zip Code 37211
Ph. (615) 883-4130

Donelson Health Spa, Inc. – Alt.
Lower Arcade – Donelson Plaza
Zip Code 37214
Ph. (615) 889-4816

Kelly Lyn Figure Salon No. 1 –
Women
3790 Nolensville Rd.
Zip Code 37211
Ph. (615) 834-5502

Kelly Lyn Figure Salon No. 3 –
Women
4004 Hillsboro Rd., Suite 234
Zip Code 37215
Ph. (615) 297-9507

Roman Health Spa – Alt.
100 Oaks Shopping Center
Thompson Center
Thompson Lane – Powell Ave.
Zip Code 37204
Ph. (615) 297-9551

**TEXAS**

**ABILENE**
Magic Mirror Figure Salon –
Women
2902 N. First St.
Zip Code 79604
Ph. (915) 677-4386

**ALICE**
Woman's World of Fitness –
Women
319 E. First Street
Zip Code 78332
Ph. (512) 668-8832

**AMARILLO**
John's Gym – Men
4311 W. 45th St.
Zip Code 79109
Ph. (806) 353-4319

Olympix U.S.A. Inc. – Dual
1619 S. Kentucky St.
Zip Code 79102
Ph. (806) 353-9834

**ARLINGTON**
National Health Studios – Women
2234 S. Collins
Zip Code 76013
Ph. (817) 265-6473

Presidents Health & Racquet
Clubs – Co-ed
2306 S. Collins
Zip Code 76014
Ph. (817) 274-7177

**ATHENS**
Shape Up Health Club – Alt.
607 E. Tyler
Zip Code 75751
Ph. (214) 675-9164

**AUSTIN**
Austin Athletic Club – Dual
9063 Research
Zip Code 78759
Ph. (512) 837-8611

New Day Health Center – Alt.
2700 Anderson Lane, No. 805
Zip Code 78757
Ph. (512) 458-2285 or 2286

Figure World of Austin – Women
1925-A Peyton Gin Rd.
Zip Code 78758
Ph. (512) 454-5891

Figure World of Austin No. 2 –
Women
South Austin – 1300 W. Ben
White
Zip Code 78704
Ph. (512) 244-4897

Figure World of Austin No. 3 –
Women
7028 Woodhollow
Zip Code 78731
Ph. (512) 346-2300

Texas Fitness Center
7045 Village Center Dr.
Zip Code 78731
Ph. (512) 346-3237

Trim & Swim Health & Beauty
Spa – Alt.
5407 Clay Ave.
Zip Code 78756
Ph. (512) 453-7251

Total Fitness Centers     Alt.
5736 Manchaca Rd.
Zip Code 78745
Ph. (512) 443-3633

Total Fitness Center     Alt.
1204 E. 38½ Street
Zip Code 78722
Ph. (512) 458-2246

**BAY CITY**
Bay City Health & Fitness Center
Alt.
2220 Avenue F
Zip Code 77414
Ph. (713) 244-2429

**BAYTOWN**
Total Fitness Center     Alt.
2137 N. Alexander
Zip Code 77520
Ph. (713) 427-5851

Total Woman Fitness Center –
Women
4312 Craigmont
Zip Code 77520
Ph. (713) 424-4509

**BEAUMONT**
Mr. Physical Fitness Nautilus
Training Center – Men
4725 Concord Rd.
Village Shopping Center
Zip Code 77702
Ph. (713) 898-0790

**BIG SPRING**
Magic Mirror Figure Salon –
Women
10 Highland Center
Zip Code 79720
Ph. (915) 263-7381

**BROWNSVILLE**
Woman's World of Fitness –
Women
3025 Boca Chica
Zip Code 78520
Ph. (512) 541-9411

**BROWNWOOD**
Magic Mirror Figure Salon –
Women
Zip Code 75801
Ph. (915) 646-1410

**BRYAN**
Nautilus of Bryan-College Station
- Men
3832 So. Texas Ave.
Zip Code 77801
Ph. (713) 846-6666

The Figure Salon     Women
3701 E. 29th
Zip Code 77801
Ph. (713) 846-3794

**BURLESON**
Magic Mirror Figure Salon –
Women
349 N.W. Renfro St.
Zip Code 76028
Ph. (817) 295-7191

**CLEAR LAKE CITY**
Magic Mirror Figure Salon –
Women
16626 Sealark Dr.
Zip Code 77058
Ph. (713) 488-8250

CLEBURNE
Magic Mirror Figure Salon —
Women
116 Williams St.
Zip Code 76031
Ph. (817) 645-6609

CLUTE
Brazosport Fitness Center, Inc.
— Men
86 Flag Lake
Zip Code 77531
Ph. (713) 297-1126

CORPUS CHRISTI
American Health Studio — Men
4154 S. Staple
Zip Code 78411
Ph. (512) 854-3113

Barbee's Executive Health Club —
Men
B-100 Guaranty Bank Plaza
Zip Code 78475
Ph. (512) 883-4459

Bradshaw's Athletic Club — Dual
4320 S. Padre Island
Zip Code 78411
Ph. (512) 851-0861

Feminique — Women
5301 Everhart
Zip Code 78411
Ph. (512) 855-4721

DALLAS
Cosmopolitan Lady — Women
5511 A Arapaho Rd.
Prestonwood Village Shopping Ctr.
Zip Code 75248
Ph. (214) 980-8009

Elegante Lady, Inc. — Women
7035 Greenville Ave.
Zip Code 75231
Ph. (214) 363-7671

Mademoiselle Spa — Women
108 Spring Valley Shopping Ctr.
Zip Code 75240
Ph. (214) 960-0966

National Health Studios — Alt.
6160 Sherry Lane
Zip Code 75225
Ph. (214) 691-1001

Presidents-First Lady Spa —
Women
3883 Turtle Creek Blvd.
Zip Code 75219
Ph. (214) 528-1650

Presidents-First Lady Spa — Alt.
539 Casa Linda Plaza
Garland Rd. & Buckner Blvd.
Zip Code 75218
Ph. (214) 247-0171

Presidents-First Lady Spa — Alt.
Metro Federal Savings Bldg.
Zip Code 75202
Ph. (214) 747-3707

DEL RIO
National Health Figure Spa —
Women
2400 Ave. F
Zip Code 78840
Ph. 775-9516

DENTON
National Health Studios — Dual
2006 University Dr.
Zip Code 76201
Ph. (817) 482-4484

FRIENDSWOOD
Elegance, A Health Fitness &
Beauty Center — Women
128 S. Friendswood Drive
Zip Code 77546
Ph. (713) 482-4484

FORT WORTH
Fort Worth Athletic Club — Dual
3900 Benbrook Hwy.
Zip Code 76116
Ph. (817) 244-0076

Gym & Trim Health & Fitness
Club — Alt.
777 W. Rosedale
Zip Code 76104
Ph. (817) 336-7162

National Health Studios — Dual
5701 Westcreek
Zip Code 76133
Ph. (817) 294-0130

Presidents-First Lady Spa
2000 Beach Street
Meadowbrook
Zip Code 76103
Ph. (817) 534-0286

GALVESTON
Figure World — Women
6209 Stewart Rd.
K-Mart Shopping Center
Zip Code 77550
Ph. (713) 744-5369

Total Fitness Center — Men
6111 Stewart Rd.
Zip Code 77551
Ph. (713) 744-0413

GARLAND
Pneuma Fitness Center — Dual
419 Walnut Park Shopping Ctr.
Zip Code 75042
Ph. (214) 494-0224

HARLINGTON
Wide World of Fitness — Women
77 Sunshine Strip Suite D-1
Zip Code 78550
Ph. (512) 452-9081

HOUSTON
Clear Lake Athletic Club — Dual
1120 Nasa Blvd., Suite 100
Zip Code 77058
Ph. (713) 333-4848

Heavenly Body Health & Fitness
Center — Women
2549 Gessner
Zip Code 77080
Ph. (713) 462-9934

Magic Mirror Figure Salon —
Women
16504 Sealark
Zip Code 77602
Ph. (713) 488-8350

Olympia Fitness & Racquetball
Club — Dual
P.O. Box 36521
Zip Code 77036
Ph. (713) 988-8787

Presidents-First Lady — Women
1709 Post Oak at San Felipe
Zip Code 77027
Ph. (713) 622-7181

Presidents-First Lady Spa — Alt.
3905-7 Bellaire Blvd.
Zip Code 77025
Ph. (713) 666-0141

Presidents-First Lady Spa — Men
9825 Katy Rd.
Zip Code 77024
Ph. (713) 467-8181

Presidents-First Lady Spa —
Women
9823 Katy Rd.
Zip Code 77024
Ph. (713) 467-8181

Presidents-First Lady Spa — Alt.
7255 Clarewood (1st Floor)
Zip Code 77036
Ph. (713) 771-8395

Presidents-First Lady Spa — Alt.
1418 Spencer Hwy.
Zip Code 77587
Ph. (713) 941-3584

Presidents-First Lady Spa — Alt.
4424 North Shepherd
Zip Code 77018
Ph. (713) 695-5824

Presidents-First Lady Spa — Dual
5215 FM 1960 West
Zip Code 77069
Ph. (713) 440-9835

Roman Health Spa — Alt.
17424 N.W. Fry. At Jones Rd.
Zip Code 77040
Ph. (712) 466-9375

Roman Health Spa — Dual
127 W. Dyna
Zip Code 77037
Ph. (712) 445-1228

Woman's World of Fitness — Alt.
5333 Antoine Dr.
Zip Code 77092
Ph. (713) 681-0637

World Wide Health Studios —
Men
2035 S. Post Oak
Zip Code 77056
Ph. (713) 622-4671

World Wide Health Studios —
Women
3920 N. Shepherd
Zip Code 77008
Ph. (713) 869-3447

World Wide Health Studios —
Women
8334 Gulf Frwy.
Zip Code 77017
Ph. (713) 644-1638

World Wide Health Studios —
Women
1035 Eastex Frwy.
Zip Code 77093
Ph. (713) 692-5903

World Wide Health Studios —
Men
8318 Gulf Frwy.
Zip Code 77017
Ph. (713) 644-3201

World Wide Health Studios —
Women
10984 Westheimer
Zip Code 77042
Ph. (713) 789-5130

World Wide Health Studios —
Women
9632 Braeswood
Zip Code 77074
Ph. (713) 777-8000

World Wide Health Studios of
Houston — Dual
P.O. Box 20328
7015 Almeda Rd.
Zip Code 77025
Ph. (713) 748-1500

HUMBLE
Roman Health Spa — Alt.
228 W. 1st
Zip Code 77338
Ph. (712) 446-0165

HURST
Presidents-First Lady Spa of
Hurst — Alt.
453 Bedford-Euless Road
Zip Code 76503
Ph. (817) 282-6774

IRVING
Irving Athletic Club — Dual
1501 W. Airport Freeway
Zip Code 75601
Ph. (214) 256-1569

Presidents-First Lady Spa — Alt.
2016 W. Grauwyler at Bradford
Zip Code 75060
Ph. (214) 259-2671

KILLEEN
Figure World — Women
223 E. Hallmark
Zip Code 76541
Ph. (817) 526-8551

Magic Mirror Figure Salon —
Women
440 Plaza Shopping Center
Zip Code 76544
Ph. (817) 526-1569

Total Fitness Center — Dual
1008 Plaza
Zip Code 76541
Ph. (817) 526-9586

LAKE JACKSON
Olympic Nautilus — Alt.
105 This Way
Zip Code 77566
Ph. (713) 297-1144

Shapely Lady Figure Salon No. 8,
Inc. — Women
458 E. Plantation
Zip Code 77566
Ph. (713) 297-7277

LEWISVILLE
National Health Studios — Dual
154 Lakeland Plaza
Zip Code 75067
Ph. 436-6548

LIBERTY
Slim & Trim Health Club
Women
2722 N. Main Street

P.O. Box 1227
Zip Code 77575
Ph. (713) 336-2862

LONGVIEW
Figure World — Women
312 Spur 63
Zip Code 75601
Ph. (214) 753-8626

Louisa Health & Beauty Resort —
Women
1210 Greenleaf
Zip Code 75601
Ph. (214) 297-2761

Magic Mirror Figure Salon —
Women
1809 W. Frank Ave.
Zip Code 75901
Ph. (713) 639-3158

LUBBOCK
Cosmopolitan Spa
5015 University Ave.
Zip Code 79412
Ph. (806) 793-8584

LUFKIN
Figure World — Women
203 No. John Redditt
Zip Code 75901
Ph. (713) 632-6668

Magic Mirror Figure Salon —
Women
1809 W. Frank Ave.
Zip Code 75901
Ph. (713) 639-3158

MARFA
el Paisano Health Spa — Alt.
207 N. Highland
Zip Code 79843
Ph. (713) 977-2780

McALLEN
Shapely Lady Figure Salon No.
10, Inc. — Women
2610 N. 10th
Zip Code 78501
Ph. (512) 687-8501

MT. PLEASANT
Slenderella — Women
401 S. Madison
Southtown Plaza
Zip Code 75455
Ph. (214) 572-3629

MIDLAND
Golden Life Fitness Center &
Racquetball Club — Dual
3200 Andrews Hwy.
Zip Code 79701
Ph. (915) 697-3223

Magic Mirror Figure Salon —
Women
Town & Country Shopping Center
Zip Code 79701
Ph. (915) 694-8863

NACOGDOCHES
Figure World — Women
1326 University Dr.
Zip Code 75961
Ph. (713) 569-7979

NEW BRAUNFELS
Figure World — Women
655 Landa
Zip Code 78139
Ph. (512) 625-7328

ODESSA
Body Shop for Women — Women
814 Nabors Lane
Zip Code 79761
Ph. (915) 333-6668

Golden Life Fitness Center
1515 N. Grandview
Zip Code 79760
Ph. (915) 367-8632

Neal's Health Fitness Club    Men
1551 N. Parkway
Zip Code 79761
Ph. (915) 337-7271

PARIS
Magic Mirror Figure Salon
Women
3552 Lamar Ave.
Zip Code 75460
Ph. (214) 785-0721

PECOS
National Health & Figure Spa -
Alt.
2028 S. Eddy
Zip Code 79772
Ph. (915) 447-2211

PLANO
Mademoiselle Spa — Women
1301 Custer, Suite 482
Zip Code 75075
Ph. (214) 867-1580

National Health Studios — Dual
1360 Parker Rd.
Zip Code 75075
Ph. (214) 596-5307

Spectrum Fitness Center
1201 N. Central Ex. 50
Zip Code 75075
Ph. (214) 424-3565

PORT ARTHUR
Cleopatra Health Spa — Women
3647 Twin City Hwy.
Jefferson City Shopping Center
Zip Code 77640
Ph. (713) 962-0274

Nautilus Fitness Center of Port
Arthur
Jefferson City Shopping Center
Zip Code 77640
Ph. (713) 962-5793

RICHARDSON
National Health Studios — Alt.
52 Richardson Heights Shopping
Center
Zip Code 75208
Ph. (214) 231-4668

Presidents-First Lady Spa — Alt.
530 W. Arapaho Rd.
Zip Code 75080
Ph. (214) 231-8251

ROSENBERG
The Fitness Factory — Alt.
1218 Herndon Drive
Zip Code 77471
Ph. (713) 342-8093

**SAN ANGELO**
Magic Mirror Figure Salon –
Women
4830 Knickerbocker Rd.
Zip Code 75901
Ph. (915) 944-1563

**SAN ANTONIO**
Figure World – Women
8102 Cross Creek
Zip Code 78218
Ph. (512) 653-9333

Figure World – Women
9401 San Pedro
Zip Code 78216
Ph. (512) 342-3226

Figure World – Women
6162 Wurzbach
Zip Code 78240
Ph. (512) 684-2533

Figure World – Women
1351 Fair Ave.
Zip Code 78223
Ph. (512) 532-3247

Figure World – Women
310 Valley Hi, Bldg. C
Zip Code 78227
Ph. (512) 673-3113

Figure World
698 SW Military Dr.
Zip Code 78221
Ph. (512) 924-7151

Figure World – Women
8023 Callaghan
Zip Code 78240
Ph. (512) 344-4564

Nautilus Fitness Center – Men
1702 S. Hackberry (at IH-10)
Zip Code 78210
Ph. (512) 534-8473

Olympic Fitness Center – Dual
4731 Rittiman Rd.
Zip Code 78218
Ph. (512) 657-2211

Trim & Swim Health & Beauty
Spa – Alt.
1335 N.W. Loop Expressway
Zip Code 78209
Ph. (512) 828-3125

Trim & Swim Health Spa – Alt.
940 Bandera Rd.
Zip Code 78228
Ph. (512) 433-8201

Trim & Swim Health Spa – Alt.
4202 San Pedro Ave.
Zip Code 78212
Ph. (512) 735-9141

**SAN MARCOS**
Figure World – Women
Ranch Road 12 and LBJ
Zip Code 78666
Ph. (512) 392-0174

**SHERMAN**
Magic Mirror Figure Salon –
Women
1907 U.S. Highway 75 North
Zip Code 75090
Ph. (214) 893-9536

National Health Studios – Alt.
3822 Frisco Rd.
Zip Code 75090
Ph. (214) 893-7418

**SPRING**
Spring-Cypress Cultural & Recre-
ational Center – Dual
723 Spring-Cypress Road
Zip Code 77373
Ph. (713) 353-5994

**TEMPLE**
Figure World – Women
4401 S. General Bruce Dr.
Town & Country Shopping Ctr.
Zip Code 76501
Ph. (817) 788-1876

Total Fitness Center
Market Place Shopping Center
Zip Code 76501
Ph. (817) 773-7694

**TEXAS CITY**
Magic Mirror Figure Salon
Women
3529 Palmer Highway
Zip Code 77590
Ph. (713) 948-3058

**TYLER**
Figure World – Women
1859 Proup Hwy.
Green Acre Shopping Center
Zip Code 75701
Ph. (214) 593-9483

**VICTORIA**
Eternal Flame Health Spa – Alt.
3003 N. Navarro St.
Zip Code 77901
Ph. (512) 573-6321

**WACO**
Figure World – Women
211 Industrial
Zip Code 76710
Ph. (817) 772-6571

Korea Taekwon-Do Academy –
Dual
3318 Franklin Center
Zip Code 76710
Ph. (817) 776-7821

Total Fitness Center – Men
430 Lake Air Dr.
Zip Code 76710
Ph. (817) 772-6140

**WAXAHACHIE**
National Health & Figure Spa –
Alt.
400 Krooger Plaza
Zip Code 75165
Ph. (214) 937-8021

**WEATHERFORD**
College Park Health Spa – Dual
144 College Park Dr.
Zip Code 76086
Ph. (817) 599-9447

**WEBSTER**
Clear Lake Athletic Club – Dual
1000 Highway 3 South
Zip Code 77598

**WHITNEY**
Figure Trim – Women
P.O. Box 1202
Downtown Whitney
Zip Code 76692
Ph. (817) 694-2706

**WICHITA FALLS**
Spa International – Alt.
3009 Garnet, Paker Square
Zip Code 76308
Ph. (817) 767-8551

# UTAH

**BOUNTIFUL**
Sophisticated Lady – Women
575 W. 2600 South
Zip Code 84010
Ph. (801) 298-3530

**KAYSVILLE**
Sophisticated Lady Fitness
Salon – Women
352 North Main
Zip Code 84037
Ph. (801) 766-2431

**LOGAN**
Athenian Health Spa – Alt.
48 N. 1st West
Zip Code 84321
Ph. (801) 753-1700

**MURRAY**
Spa Fitness Center – Fual
155 East 6100 South
Zip Code 84017
Ph. (801) 268-0606

**NORTH SALT LAKE**
Larry Scott's Health & Racquet
Club – Dual
410 No. Main St.
Zip Code 84054
Ph. (801) 295-9421

**OGDEN**
Feminine Fitness World – Women
4387 Harrison Blvd.
Zip Code 84403
Ph. (801) 479-0070

Lady Fitness – Women
145 N. Washington Blvd.
P.O. Box 2465
Zip Code 84404
Ph. (801) 399-4474

Sophisticated Lady Fitness Salon
– Women
2074 Harrison Blvd.
Zip Code 84401
Ph. (801) 394-9481

Spa Fitness Center – Dual
3354 Harrison Blvd.
Zip Code 84403
Ph. (801) 621-6350

**OREM**
Spa Fitness Center – Dual
703 South State
Zip Code 84057
Ph. (801) 225-7750

**ROY**
American Health & Sports Center
– Dual
5385 S. 1950 West
Zip Code 84067
Ph. (801) 773-6220

SALT LAKE CITY
Sophisticated Lady Figure Salon
— Women
2120 S. 1300 East, No. 102
Zip Code 84106

Sophisticated Lady of Salt Lake,
Inc. — Women
Hillside Shopping Center
2400 East 7000 South Street
Zip Code 84121
Ph. (801) 943-LADY

Spa Fitness Center — Dual
4700 Highland Dr.
Zip Code 84117
Ph. (801) 278-2846

Spa Fitness Center — Dual
1033 East 21st South
Zip Code 84106
Ph. (801) 484-8766

Spa La'Fem — Women
3924 S. Highland Dr.
Zip Code 84117
Ph. (801) 278-4461

SANDY
Spa La'Fem — Women
9460 S. Union Square
Zip Code 84070
Ph. (801) 571-0250

Spa La'Fem — Women
9484 S. 7th East Union Square
Zip Code 84070
Ph. (801) 581-0250

TREMONTON
Riviera Health Spa — Dual
113 W. Main
Zip Code 84337
Ph. (801) 257-7466

W. JORDAN
Spa La'Fem — Women
7866 S. Redwood Rd.
Zip Code 84084
Ph. (801) 566-8255

WEST VALLEY
3581 Market Street
Zip Code 84119
Ph. (801) 966-1388

# VIRGINIA

ALEXANDRIA
Atrium Health Club — Dual
277 S. Washington St.
Zip Code 22314
Ph. (703) 549-5444

Mt. Vernon Square Nautilus —
Dual
2915 Arlington Dr.
Zip Code 22306
Ph. (703) 660-6878

Slender Lady Figure Salon
6218 Little River Turnpike
Zip Code 22312
Ph. (703) 941-0686

Spa Lady — Women
255-257 S. Van Dorn St.
Zip Code 22304
Ph. (703) 823-5252

ARLINGTON
Fun and Fitness, Inc. — Dual
3321 Lee Highway
Zip Code 22207
Ph. (703) 524-6660

Lookin' Good — Women
2052 N. Albermarie St.
Zip Code 22207
Ph. (703) 276-9400

BURKE
Burke Nautilus — Dual
9566 Burke Rd.
Zip Code 22015
Ph. (703) 425-5115

CHARLOTTESVILLE
Holiday Health & Racquet Club —
Dual
475 Westfield Road
Zip Code 22901
Ph. (804) 973-1307

CHESAPEAKE
Holiday Health & Fitness Center
3124 Western Drive
Popular Hill Plaza

Miss Universe Spa & Beauty Resort — Women
831 St. Lawrence Dr.
Zip Code 23325
Ph. (804) 543-1631

DALE CITY
Lookin' Good — Women
4323 Dale Blvd., Center Plaza
Zip Code 22193
Ph. (703) 680-4909

DANVILLE
Danville Fitness Center — Women
Kings Fairground Plaza
Piney Forest Rd.
Zip Code 24541
Ph. (804) 797-5800

Nautilus Fitness Center — Dual
3304 Riverside Drive
Riverside Shopping Center
Zip Code 24541
Ph. (804) 799-1397 (Women)
Ph. (804) 799-1424 (Men)

FAIRFAX
Nautilus Fitness Center — Dual
3131 Draper Drive
Zip Code 22031
Ph. (703) 691-1180

Spa Lady — Women
10366 Democracy
Zip Code 22030
Ph. (703) 273-7955

Fitness World — Women
10681 Braddock Rd.
Zip Code 22032
Ph. (703) 591-2550

Lookin' Good — Women
11706L Fair Oaks Mall
Zip Code 22033
Ph. (703) 385-3776

FALLS CHURCH
Nautilus Fitness Factory — Dual
6184 B Arlington Blvd.
Zip Code 22044
Ph. (703) 533-1242

Spa Lady — Women
6769 Wilson Blvd.
Plaza 7 Shopping Center
Zip Code 22044
Ph. (703) 533-0462

FREDERICKSBURG
Spa Health Club — Alt.
1032 Warrenton Rd.
Old Forge Plaza
Zip Code 22401
Ph. (703) 371-6235

HAMPTON
Holiday Health & Fitness Center
2007 Cunningham Drive
Riverdale Shopping Center
Zip Code 23666

Nautilus Fitness Center of Hamp-
ton — Dual
2326 W. Mercury Blvd.
Todd Center
Zip Code 23666
Ph. (804) 838-2020

HOPEWELL
Old Diminion Nautilus/Hopewell
— Alt.
Bldg. 14, Lee Plaza
Zip Code 23860
Ph. (804) 541-1856

LYNCHBERG
Nautilus Super Fitness — Dual
3 Wadsworth St.
Zip Code 24502
Ph. (804) 528-5911

MANASSAS
Fun and Fitness, Inc. — Dual
8300 Sudley Rd.
Zip Code 22110
Ph. (703) 361-2104

NEWPORT NEWS
The Health Club — Alt.
6120 Jefferson Ave.
Zip Code 23605
Ph. (703) 826-0411

Health Club Spa — Alt.
14104 Warwick Blvd.
Zip Code 23602
Ph. (703) 874-1915

Miss Universe Spa Salon — Women
300 Oyster Point Road
Zip Code 23602
Ph. (804) 877-1344

NORFOLK
Holiday Health & Fitness Center
7401 Grandy St.
Ward's Corner
Zip Code 23505

Nautilus Fitness Center — Dual
80 Janaf Shopping Center
Zip Code 23502
Ph. (804) 461-5511

The Garden Spa & Health Club,
Ltd. — Alt.
7924 Chesapeake Blvd.
Zip Code 23518
Ph. (804) 480-3737

NORTON
Doug's Fitness World, Inc. — Dual
1763 Park Ave. SW
Zip Code 24273
Ph. (703) 679-4860

**PETERSBURG**
Old Dominion Nautilus of Petersburg — Co-ed
2557 South Crater Rd.
Zip Code 23803
Ph. (804) 861-3284

**PORTSMOUTH**
Nautilus Fitness Center — Alt.
5911 High St. West
Zip Code 23703
Ph. (804) 484-4355

**RICHMOND**
Nautilus Fitness Center — Co-ed
1538 Paraham Road
Zip Code 23219
Ph. (804) 747-9493

Nautilus Fitness Centers — Co-ed
1011 E. Main Street
Zip Code 23219
Ph. (804) 643-6587

Nautilus Fitness Clinic — Alt.
6510 Hull Street Rd.
Zip Code 23235
Ph. (804) 276-6717

World-Wide Health Spa —
Women
2833 Hathaway Rd.
Stratford Hills
Zip Code 23225
Ph. (804) 272-7581

World Wide Health Spa —
Women
4951 Nine Mile Rd.
Eastgate Shopping Center
Zip Code 23223
Ph. (804) 222-2204

World Wide Health Studios of
Richmond — Dual
4248 Parham Rd.
Ridge Shopping Center
Zip Code 23229
Ph. (703) 282-4248

**ROANOKE**
Cosmopolitan Spa International,
Inc. — Alt.
4351 Avenhan Avenue Extension
Zip Code 24014
Ph. (703) 989-6118

**SOUTH BOSTON**
Halifax Athletic Club — Dual
4110 Centerville Area
Zip Code 24582
Ph. (804) 572-3919

**SPRINGFIELD**
Nautilus Fitness Center — Dual
6715 Backlick Road
Zip Code 22150
Ph. (703) 455-2704

Spa Lady — Women
6230-20 Rolling Rd.
Zip Code 22152
Ph. (703) 451-3302

**STERLING**
Capitol Courts Club Nautilus —
Dual
308 Glenn Dr.
Zip Code 22170
Ph. (703) 430-0668

Nautilus Fitness Center — Dual
91 H.F. Byrd Hwy.
Zip Code 22170
Ph. (703) 450-5157

**SUFFOLK**
Nautilus Conditioning Center —
Dual
701 E. Pinner St.
Zip Code 23434
Ph. (804) 934-3215

**VIRGINIA BEACH**
Empress Spa Lady — Women
825 Chimney Hill
Zip Code 23452
Ph. (804) 463-0349

Holiday Health & Fitness Centers
4716 Virginia Beach Blvd.
Zip Code 23462

Holiday Health & Fitness Center
1284 Laskin Road
Zip Code 23451

Miss Universe Spa Salon — Women
2126 Great Neck Square
Zip Code 23462
Ph. (804) 424-5298

Miss Universe Spa Salon — Women
995 Providence Square Shopping
Center
Zip Code 23462
Ph. (804) 424-5298

Nautilus Fitness Center of Virginia Beach — Men
507 Hilltop Plaza Shopping Ctr.
Zip Code 23451
Ph. (804) 422-3636

Nautilus Fitness Center — Alt.
1033 Independence Blvd.
Haygood Shopping Center
Zip Code 23455
Ph . (804) 464-5555

Scandinavian Health Club — Alt.
3464 Holland Road
Zip Code 23185
Ph. (804) 468-3605

**WILLIAMSBURG**
Nautilus of Williamsburg — Dual
1270 Richmond Rd.
Zip Code 23185
Ph. (804) 220-3180

**WOODBRIDGE**
Fun and Fitness, Inc. — Dual
14412 Jeff Davis Hwy.
Zip Code 22191
Ph. (703) 494-5126

Spa Lady — Women
13995 Jefferson Davis Hwy.
Zip Code 22191
Ph. (703) 491-2138

# WASHINGTON

**ABERDEEN**
Nautilus Fitness Center — Co-ed
311 W. Market
Zip Code 98520
Ph. (206) 533-6115

**BELLEVUE**
Family Fitness Center — Alt.
1505 NE 140th
Zip Code 98005
Ph. (209) 641-5615

**BELLINGHAM**
Family Fitness Center — Alt.
Bellingham Mall
Zip Code 98225
Ph. (209) 676-0700

**BREMERTON**
Family Fitness Center — Alt.
5600 Kitsap Way
Zip Code 98310
Ph. (209) 479-0610

**BURIEN**
Family Fitness Center — Alt.
156 SW 156th
Zip Code 98149
Ph. (209) 242-9641

**CHEHALIS**
New Profile Spa — Alt.
1793 Kresky Ave.
Zip Code 98532
Ph. (206) 748-3381

**COLLEGE PLACE**
NuLife Health Spa — Co-ed
418-B So. College
Zip Code 99324
Ph. (509) 529-3361

**FEDERAL WAY**
Family Fitness Center — Alt.
1430 S. 330th St.
Zip Code 98003
Ph. (209) 838-3860

Pacific West Sport & Racquet
Clubs, Inc.
32818 1st Avenue South
Zip Code 98003
Ph. (206) 927-3312

Total Woman Health Studio —
Women
32065 Pacific Hwy.
Zip Code 98003
Ph. (206) 839-9310

**GIG HARBOR**
Pacific West Sport & Racquet
Clubs, Inc.
2002 36th Street NW
Zip Code 98335
Ph. (206) 272-9865 or 858-9115

**KENNEWICK**
Lady Fitness — Women
3180 W. Clearwater
Zip Code 99336
Ph. (509) 735-7594

**OLYMPIA**
Capitol Fitness and Recreation
Center — Men & Women
8901 Martin Way
Zip Code 98506
Ph. (206) 491-1462

**PORT ANGELES**
Fitness America/Olympic Fitness
— Dual
Ridgeview Center
1005 E. Front St.
Zip Code 98362
Ph. (206) 452-7878

**SEATTLE**
Gentlemen's Gym — Dual
18915 16th South
Zip Code 98148
Ph. (206) 244-3010

The Body Seattle — Men
1501 12th Ave.
Zip Code 98102
Ph. (206) 329-2639

Family Fitness Center — Alt.
15220 Aurora North
Zip Code 98121
Ph. (209) 367-5120

Family Fitness Center — Alt.
2306 6th Ave.
Zip Code 98121
Ph. (209) 624-3122

In-Trim Health Studio — Alt.
6423 Fauntleroy Way SW
Zip Code 98136
Ph. (206) 937-7026

Olympic Racquet & Health Club
— Dual
5301 Leary Ave., NW
Zip Code 98107
Ph. (206) 789-5010

Washington Conditioning Club —
Dual
15281-B Fourth Ave.
Zip Code 98101
Ph. (206) 682-4036

**SPOKANE**
Family Fitness Center — Alt.
9233 E. Montgomery
Zip Code 99206
Ph. (509) 926-6268

Lady Fitness — Women
14214 E. Sprague
Zip Code 99216
Ph. (509) 928-2275

**TACOMA**
Family Fitness Center — Alt.
3338 S. 78th
Zip Code 98489
Ph. (509) 475-1041

**YAKIMA**
Family Fitness Center — Alt.
1211 W. Lincoln Ave.
Zip Code 98902
Ph. (509) 248-5825

**WASHINGTON, D.C.**

Fun & Fitness, Inc. — Dual
L'Enfant Plaza, SW
Promenade Level, Suite 710
Zip Code 20024
Ph. (202) 554-8801

Nautilus Fitness Centers — Dual
1901 Pennsylvania Ave., NW
Zip Code 20006
Ph. (202) 887-0760

**WEST VIRGINIA**

**FAIRMONT**
Country Club Health Spa — Alt.
1499 Locust Ave.
Zip Code 26554
Ph. (304) 366-1962

**HUNTINGTON**
Nautilus Sports and Fitness Cen-
ter — Dual
919 Sixth Ave.
Zip Code 25701
Ph. (304) 523-5555

Pam's Fitness Centers — Women
2640 5th Avenue
Zip Code 27502
Ph. (304) 525-5006

**KEYSER**
Perky Health Spa — Alt.
126 Spring Street
Zip Code 26726
Ph. (304) 788-5431

**WISCONSIN**

**FOX POINT**
Vic Tanny Health Club — Alt.
7950 N. Port Washington Rd.
Zip Code 53217
Ph. (414) 352-1910

**GREEN BAY**
Wisconsin Athletic Club — Alt.
1134 S. Military Avenue
Zip Code 54304
Ph. (414) 494-9501

**GREENDALE**
Vic Tanny Health & Racquet
Club — Dual
5474 S. 76th St.
Zip Code 53129
Ph. (414) 421-9250

**GREENFIELD**
Vic Tanny Health Spa — Alt.
4200 S. 76th St., Spring Mall
Zip Code 53219
Ph. (414) 327-1810

Vic Tanny Health Spa — Women
400 W. Silver Springs Dr.
Zip Code 53217
Ph. (414) 964-6400

**JANESVILLE**
Continental Spa of Janesville,
Inc. — Alt.
2100 E. Milwaukee St.
Fairview Mall
Zip Code 53545
Ph. (608) 257-1300

Vic Tanny — Dual
26 Schroeder Ct.
Zip Code 53711
Ph. (608) 273-2110

**MILWAUKEE**
Vic Tanny Health Club — Women
3333 S. 27th St., Southgate
Zip Code 53215
Ph. (414) 671-4100

**RACINE**
Vic Tanny Health Clubs — Alt.
5420 So. Lakeshore Rd.
Zip Code 53404
Ph. (414) 552-9513

**WAUWATOSA**
Vic Tanny Health Club — Women
2717 N. Mayfair Rd.
Zip Code 53222
Ph. (414) 774-3000

Vic Tanny Health & Racquet
Club — Dual
2930 North 117th Street
Zip Code 53222
Ph. (414) 475-0777

V.I.P. Physical Health Club, Inc.
— Dual
2500 N. Mayfair Rd.
Zip Code 53226
Ph. (414) 257-3878

**WYOMING**

**CASPER**
Nautilus Fitness Center — Dual
4080 S. Poplar
Zip Code 82601
Ph. (307) 266-4398

# About the Author

David Francko has spent most of his life in the midwest, where health clubs are popular, especially during the winter months when outdoor activities are restricted to cross-country skiing and snow shoveling. He received a Ph.D. in Physiological Limnology (the study of chemical and biological properties of fresh water) at Michigan State University after which he completed post-doctoral work at the W.K. Kellogg biological station of Michigan State before moving to Stillwater, Oklahoma. He is now an assistant professor of Botany at Oklahoma State University. Francko enjoys a game of racquetball at the local university gym to supplement his weight training program and is a certified scuba diver.

# Recommended Reading

**Warm-Up/Warm-Down Activities and Aerobics**

*Aerobics,* by Kenneth Cooper, Bantam Books, 1968.

*Jogging,* by William Bowerman and W.E. Harris, Grosset and Dunlap, 1967.

*Jogging for Fitness and Weight Control,* by Frederick B. Roby and Russell P. Davis, W.B. Saunders Company, 1970.

*New Exercises for Runners,* by the editors of *Runner's World,* Anderson World, Inc., 1975.

*Stretching,* by Bob Anderson, published by the author, Fullerton, California, 1975.

*The Runner's World Yoga Book,* by Jean Couch and Nell Weaver, Anderson World, Inc., Mountain View, California, 1979.

**Strength Training**

*Arnold's Bodyshaping for Women,* by Arnold Schwarzenneger, Simon and Schuster, 1980.

*Arnold: The Education of a Bodybuilder,* by Arnold Schwarzenneger and Douglas Kent Hall, Simon and Schuster, 1977.

*Complete Weight Training Book,* by Bill Reynolds, Anderson World, Inc., 1976.

*Getting Strong,* by Kathryn Lance, Bobs-Merrill Co., 1978.

*Inside Weight Training for Women,* by Doris Barrileax and Jim Murray, Contemporary Books, 1978.

*The Gold's Gym Book of Strength Training for Athletes,* by Ken Sprague, J.P. Tarcher, 1979.

*The Runner's World Strength Training Book,* by Edwin Sobey, Anderson World, Inc., 1981.

**Miscellaneous and Nutrition**

*Dear Dr. Jock . . . The People's Guide to Sports and Fitness,* by David C. Bachman, M.D. and Marilynn Preston, E.P. Dutton, 1980.

*Nutrition and Athletic Performance,* by Ellington Darden, Borden Publishing Co., 1976.

*Nutrition and the Athlete,* by Joseph J. Morello and Richard J. Turchetti, D. Van Nostrand Reinhold Co., 1975.

*The Runner's World Indoor Exercise Book,* by Richard Benyo and Rhonda Provost, Anderson World, Inc., 1981.

*The Sports Medicine Book,* by Gabe Mirkin, M.D. and Marshall Hoffman, Little, Brown, and Co., 1978.